Breast Cancer?
Let Me Check My Schedule!

Breast Cancer?

EDITED BY

*Peggy McCarthy and
Jo An Loren*

◈

with a foreword by
Erma Bombeck

Let Me Check My Schedule!

CONTRIBUTORS

Donna Cederberg
Daria Davidson
Joy Edwards
Carol Hebestreit
Betsy Lambert
Amy Langer
Cathy Masamitsu
Sally Snodgrass
Carol Stack
Carol Washington

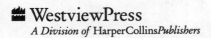 WestviewPress
A Division of HarperCollins*Publishers*

Copyright © 1997 by Westview Press, A Division of HarperCollins Publishers, Inc.

Published in 1997 in the United States of America by Westview Press, 5500 Central Avenue, Boulder, Colorado 80301-2877, and in the United Kingdom by Westview Press, 12 Hid's Copse Road, Cumnor Hill, Oxford OX2 9JJ

A CIP catalog record for this book is available from the Library of Congress.
ISBN 0–8133-3431-4 (hc) — ISBN 0–8133-3393-8 (pbk)

Design by Jane Raese

The paper used in this publication meets the requirements of the American National Standard for Permanence of Paper for Printed Library Materials Z39.48-1984.

10   9   8   7   6   5   4   3   2   1

To all the women—
past, present, and future—
who face the diagnosis of breast cancer

and in memory of
Donna Cederberg, who died June 4, 1995
and Joy Edwards, who died May 25, 1997

Contents

Foreword

ERMA BOMBECK

I DO NOT KNOW NOR HAVE I EVER MET the ten women who authored this book. But we share a common bond. All of us were watching our prime-time lives pass by when a voice announced, "We interrupt this life to bring you cancer." We didn't even have time to turn the dial.

I have read a hundred books on breast cancer—war stories of women who did battle with the most frightening adversary in their lives. But *Breast Cancer? Let Me Check My Schedule!* is different. These are the personal stories of ten women, all over thirty, who pursue careers outside their homes. They were part of a project conducted by McCarthy Medical Marketing and Innovative Medical Education Consortium when they discovered that these women reacted differently to cancer than other women. The way they accepted their diagnosis, the decisions they made, their approach to therapy, and the way they coped all reflected their experience in the workplace.

I wanted to be a part of this book mostly because of the title. It fit me to a tee. I too am a working woman complete with a little calendar that tells me when to have a headache. If it isn't penciled in, I don't have one. On April 23, 1992, under "Things To Do Today" I jotted down "radical mastectomy, noon."

I was a lot like Amy in the book, who, when her gynecologist warned her that lumps in her breast suggested a mammogram, got dressed, added this item to her Filofax under "medium level priority" item number eleven, and went back to the office.

When a woman is busy with a career, there is something really intrusive about cancer. Anything is intrusive that doesn't have an appointment. It doesn't fit in the schedule. It doesn't enrich your qualifications. It looks out of place on your résumé. I never wanted to be a poster child for cancer. It isn't that I don't want to help other women get through their ordeal. It has to do with the fact that I've worked twenty-eight years trying to get people to laugh at themselves. I don't want to go out of this world leaving a legacy of people with sad eyes who say, "You know, for the last three years, Erma Bombeck's columns have had a right-breasted feeling to them, don't you think?"

The George Burns line "I can't go yet, I'm booked" is a universal one in this book. The same drive that catapulted these women to superwoman status kicks in with cancer. The more demands cancer makes on them, the busier they get. They thrive on stress. It's exhausting, but it's invigorating. They have to ask themselves, did stress play a role in their disease?

There is no answer.

And yet, the focus that could be dangerous to your health is the same one that gets us through it. It may not be business as usual—but it's still business. Without deadlines to occupy my mind, maybe I wouldn't have crumbled—but everyone around me would.

We are women who no longer have control over what we are going to feel like, what they're going to do to us, and when they're going to do it. (We don't even know who "they" are.) But we have control over our work. And it feels good.

As I read this book I was hoping it would address the one emotion that all cancer patients rarely speak about: the uncertainty of our future. It did. We are a unique group who has been allowed to face our mortality, and oddly enough, it has made us better people for it. There isn't a survivor who doesn't admit she has changed.

We learn quickly how to deal with our fears and our anger. We no longer take anything for granted. Our priorities change. We live our lives on its terms—not ours.

Cancer is not doable without humor. I mean it. The note from my good friend Dear Abby who said, "So, you lost a hooter. Big deal!" (Is she Iowa, or what!) The woman who sent me a card reading, "When life gives you a bunch of lemons—stuff 'em in your bra." My dental technician, whom I asked after my mastectomy, "Do you see anything different about me?" and she said, "You changed the color of your hair." The interim cotton prosthesis a nurse gave me that prompted me to observe, "I've got bigger dust balls under my bed."

I've heard women say, "I can't read cancer books. They're downers." *Breast Cancer? Let Me Check My Schedule!* is not a downer. How could it be when you enter the lives of these ten women who triumph over an invasion of their bodies. These are women with drive and purpose who aren't ready to give up. Cancer? It's a full week. I'll have my people call your people and set something up.

⨠⨠

Erma Bombeck was diagnosed with breast cancer in 1992. Shortly after, she was diagnosed with adult polycystic kidney disease. She died on April 23, 1996, from complications suffered following a kidney transplant.

Preface

THE DIAGNOSIS OF BREAST CANCER is traumatic and terrifying to any woman. But to a woman who has struggled and worked hard to achieve success in her profession, the diagnosis brings even more profound hardships. Not only is she forced to accommodate the effects of the disease and its treatment into her life, but she must also find time for all that the diagnosis entails, in a schedule already full to capacity with life's commitments, both personal *and* professional.

During the past several years, we at McCarthy Medical Marketing (MMM) and Innovative Medical Education Consortium (IMEC) have been involved in the development of major educational programs about breast cancer. As part of these programs we have conducted numerous focus groups and interviews with breast cancer survivors. We discovered that professional women's coping styles are unique. Their decision-making processes, acceptance of their diagnoses, approach to therapy, and approach to living with breast cancer are different. As these differences became more apparent, an idea for a book took shape—a book that would identify these different coping styles and present them in a way that could benefit other women while providing a learning opportunity for health-care professionals who treat, and are often stressed by, this "different" kind of patient.

Unlike thirty, twenty, or even ten years ago, most of the more than 182,000 women newly diagnosed with breast cancer will be working women. Many will be professional women who have consciously chosen careers that require high levels of skill, special training, and a commitment of time and energy. All the contributors to this book are women accustomed to controlling all aspects of their lives. They are committed to their careers.

In 1992, MMM and IMEC approached the Wellcome Oncology group of Burroughs Wellcome Co. with our idea for a book. Wellcome Oncology agreed to provide funding to gather ten professional women for a five-day retreat to discuss the various issues that affected their coping styles. Wellcome Oncology also provided funds for a guest editor and a portion of our staff time. Hundreds of additional staff hours and the actual printing of the book were contributed by MMM and IMEC as a labor of love and as a commitment to this very exciting and worthwhile project. We believe this project exemplifies the best kind of collaboration among big and small businesses, for-profit and not-for-profit organizations, and individuals. IMEC chose to publish the book—the first, we hope, of many similar projects—and to donate 50 percent of the proceeds of the first edition of the book, after expenses, to breast cancer education. The other 50 percent was to be distributed by Wellcome Oncology to further the cause of breast cancer advocacy.

The staff members of MMM and IMEC feel very fortunate that all of the ten women who were invited to participate as contributors to *Breast Cancer? Let Me Check My Schedule!* were excited enough about the project to interrupt their scheduled commitments to share their personal lives with us, and with you. This has been an extraordinary experience for all of us. We and the contributors got to know one another in ways that some of us had never imagined and expressed feelings that many of us had never before put into words. The friendship and regard we hold for these women and that they hold for one another are fashioned of deep respect and love.

The contributors were selected because they represent a cross section of lifestyles, ages, ethnic backgrounds, geographic locations, and professions. Some we met in our focus groups or interviews; others were referred to us through major cancer support organizations throughout the United States. Despite their diversity, they share many attributes, including:

- a desire to play an active role in any decision made about their treatment and care
- an insistence that they be treated by health professionals as intelligent, capable partners in the decision-making process
- a constant curiosity about and a need to research and understand every aspect of their breast cancer and care, often challenging their health-care teams with suggestions for new, experimental approaches to therapy
- a desire and need to use their personal experiences with breast cancer to help other women with the same diagnosis

Nine of the contributors have been married at least once, and nine have also been divorced at least once. Six had children before their diagnoses, and one had her first child after her diagnosis and treatment. All of the six who had children at the time of diagnosis have been single parents at one time or another. Four have at least one daughter, three have sons, while one has both daughters and sons. Six of the women were in relationships at the time of their diagnoses, and four of them were married. One contributor's husband died shortly after her diagnosis, and two others' relationships ended by choice. One contributor who was married ended that marriage shortly after her diagnosis and began a new marriage a short time later. Three contributors began new relationships after their diagnoses and remain very committed to those relationships.

Because of the limited size of the group, we were not able to include women from all ethnic groups, professions, and lifestyles. None of the contributors are under the age of thirty, though we know there are many women in their twenties who have been diagnosed with breast cancer. Following the retreat, our staff interviewed women with breast cancer who were in categories we know were not represented by this group of contributors. Some interviewees fit our definition of "professional" and others did not. Some of the information from these interviews is included here.

All of the contributors are accustomed to and fully capable of making life choices and are confident, capable individuals. All deal with many complex issues in both their personal and professional lives and fully expect to continue doing so, leading full, active lives just as they did before their diagnoses. They all want to maintain their busy schedules, which include working long hours on the job, giving attention and time to family and other loved ones, and devoting time to various avocations that include volunteer work, civic and church activities, and hobbies. The growing need in busy, professional women for control and choice, coupled with changes in health-care delivery in the United States, will lead to many challenges for the health-care system and its practitioners over the next decade. Women with breast cancer, especially professional women, have become leaders in the patient advocacy movement, modeled gratefully on the actions of the many gay men and others who have worked so hard for patients' rights in HIV treatment. We believe strongly that these contributors represent the "tip of the iceberg" in the movement to improve the understanding and care of women with breast cancer.

For all ten contributors, the diagnosis of breast cancer was a major blow because—in addition to the medical treatment and physical changes they underwent—it interrupted their busy, active, and fulfilled lives. It was this aspect of their situations that inspired our administrative assistant to suggest the title of this book, *Breast Cancer? Let Me Check My Schedule!*

This book provides an inventive combination of information sources—direct quotations from the contributors, editorial interpretation of the contributors' thoughts and feelings, bulleted tips summarizing the contributors' major insights, and brief summaries of relevant, recently published articles in the area of breast cancer research. The book can provide a source of information and support for all women facing breast cancer but, in particular, for that unique group of professional women with breast cancer. It is also intended to provide health-care professionals with insight into what makes this group of women "different," and, in turn, to enhance their relationships with them. We especially want to reach the thousands of nurses and oncology nurse specialists who work with the hundreds of thousands of women with breast cancer each year, and who exert a tremendous amount of influence on the quality of care these women receive.

It is the contributors' and our wish that you, whether professional woman, health-care provider, family member, or friend, will turn to these pages again and again for inspiration, knowledge, and hope.

Peggy McCarthy
Executive Director
Innovative Medical Education Consortium, Inc.
President
McCarthy Medical Marketing, Inc.

Acknowledgments

WE ARE GRATEFUL for the contributions of the following people in the development of this book. Jan Tanner and Carlin Lockee for early manuscript development; Susan McCarthy for scientific research; and Mark White, Charlene Pennington, Molly Burkhart, and Carena Thompson for invaluable administrative assistance.

P.M. and J.A.L.

About the Contributors

"Cancer is a crisis in the true meaning of the [word in] Chinese . . . , which is composed of two characters, one meaning danger and the other opportunity."
—*David Spiegel*

We are ten professional women who have faced the diagnosis of breast cancer. Being diagnosed with breast cancer had an impact on our professional lives like nothing we have ever experienced. The title of this book, *Breast Cancer? Let Me Check My Schedule!*, reflects one of the first and most stressful reactions we all had upon hearing we had breast cancer. All of us have friends or know of other women who have also heard this diagnosis, and we recognized the disruption it caused in their lives. We had no idea how we could maintain our busy schedules and fit in all the medical care we knew we would need, but we knew that somehow we would have to do so.

Though all ten of us were asked to gather for a five-day retreat to organize this book, only eight were able to attend; one was recovering from a very recent stem-cell transplant and joined us by speakerphone, and one had a previous commitment to speak at a meeting about breast cancer. Because of weather and time constraints, she was unable to join us even by speakerphone. All ten of us were involved in the development of this book, and all of our stories are represented here. Most of us were strangers to one another, but it took very little time to get to know and feel comfortable with one another. The five-day retreat was spent talking about our diagnoses and treatment and identifying what we wanted others in our situation to know both about breast cancer and how we deal with it. Issues came up that we hadn't even realized were important until we faced them in our group—then we discovered they were not only important, but critical. We shared with each other the many humorous moments we had each encountered, and laughed, knowing that humor is the shell that protected us so many times through this ordeal. We also cried. We acted as catalysts for one another and were able to clearly define some of our major problems and concerns, as well as some of the ways we have found for dealing with this burden.

The most effective way we know to convey this information to you is to let you participate as a member, albeit a silent one, of our group. This book is loosely organized around the issues we identified as being of major importance to us. We have supplemented the narrative with current research studies.

We assume that you have been recently diagnosed with breast cancer and are beginning your fact-finding efforts, or that you are a partner, friend, or relative of someone diagnosed with breast cancer. Much of what we say in this book will complement the information you have collected. We want you to know about problems that arose for us and will, we suspect, arise for you. Chances are you will not find this information in any other resource. We wish we could all get together to talk with you personally, but as that is impossible, we'll just have to "book" it.

If you are a health-care professional—oncologist, oncology nurse, surgeon or radiologist, or another member of a health-care team who works with women who have breast cancer—we sincerely hope that you will read this book because much of what we have learned involves you. We appeal to you to read our words and better understand our needs, for we will demand more information, more answers, different schedules, and extra accommodation because we, like you, lead busy lives that involve commitments that we must and intend to meet. We ask that you consider us colleagues, for we are your corporate executives, your attorneys, your real estate agents, your educators, and your fellow health-care professionals. Some of the issues we faced became nonissues because you helped us find resolutions; other issues became problems because you lacked understanding about who we are and what was required of us when this most difficult of all tasks was added to our already overburdened schedules. Some of you were wonderful at helping us meet our other life commitments, but many of you still need to learn to be flexible—and to learn to really listen to and hear what your patients, especially the women, are saying.

So that you may have a better understanding of who and what we are, we present the following personal sketches—sketches that provide brief descriptions of our careers, the status of our diseases, and a glimpse of a typical day in each of our lives. The table following our stories provides a brief overview of our medical history.

Donna Cederberg: I am a master's-trained nurse and hold a management position with Burroughs Wellcome Co. in Research Triangle Park, North Carolina. I was diagnosed with breast cancer in 1990, when I was thirty-six years old, at which time I had a lumpectomy to remove a two- to three-centimeter tumor. The surgery revealed that it was an infiltrating ductal cancer; the nodes were negative. I elected to have aggressive chemotherapy. I was disease-free for two and one-half years. Then, in 1993, I found that the cancer had metastasized to my bones. I underwent hormone therapy (at this time, they call me a "hormone responder") and three weeks of radiation to my spine. I suffered a collapsed fracture of my L5 vertebra. My lower back has since healed, but I still endure spinal pain every day. In February 1994, I began chemotherapy with Cytoxan, 5-FU, and Adriamycin in preparation for a stem-cell transplant scheduled for May 1994. I'm lucky because transplantation technology has progressed rapidly, and rather than having bone marrow removed from one of my large bones in a quite painful procedure, I will be able to have a stem-cell transplant. A stem-cell transplant involves getting a number of injections of growth hormones to stimulate my marrow to produce more stem cells, followed by three days of being connected to a machine that will separate out the immature cells, or stem cells, from my blood. After the stem cells are collected, the procedure will be like a bone marrow transplant.

Of all of us who attended the retreat, I am the youngest. I was experiencing a good deal of back pain, so I arranged to have a sofa in the meeting room, on which I had to spend much of the five days. My prognosis is scary—especially for those in the group who have not had a recurrence. I tried to be completely honest, and I am not shy. As the others can attest, I felt it was important to speak candidly about my anger, fear, concerns, and frustrations.

For me a typical day starts early. Mornings are my best time! I awake refreshed after eight or nine hours of sleep.

Today, I feel no pain. I have a wonderful relationship with my husband, Mark. Mornings are special for us— quiet time to think about our day. This morning I wonder what I can do to keep joy in my life, exuberance in my outlook, and determination in my soul. I think, even with this diagnosis of metastatic disease, I can have a healthy life today! Cancer will not prevent me from having peace of mind, unconditional love, independence, and lots of laughter. I will connect directly with life today and not merely with its reflection. Mark and I commute to work together, so I get dropped at the front of my building and am quickly caught up in the rush of over one thousand of my company employees coming to work. I was recently promoted to administrator, supervising fifteen people, in the Medical Division of Burroughs Wellcome Co., where numerous new drugs are under investigation. My phone is ringing when I walk into my office, and it doesn't stop for the rest of the day. I move from telephone calls about canceled site visits and a new drug for herpes to conferences on computer problems. By now it is 11:00 A.M., and I call to schedule another appointment with my doctor; I get angry when I am kept on hold for fifteen minutes for laboratory results. I decide it's time to schedule a massage. Today, I hear from my brother, who shares a joke with me. Mark calls just to "check in." I turn down an invitation for lunch with two friends—I just don't feel like telling the story again. This afternoon I deal with budgets, professional journal articles, and performance evaluations. My back begins to ache. I have always worked ten or more hours a day, but I cannot do that today. I believe that pain is the ultimate challenge. It's hard to remember that the good times are richer against this background of sorrow. Mark picks me up at 4:00 P.M. to go home to my bed to rest before dinner. We share the details of our day over dinner and a good bottle of wine. Our evening mirrors the simplicity of our lives now: Mark cooks, I clean. Laughter ends even the saddest commentary. At 8:00 P.M. we are reading in bed. I feel so fortunate to have Mark as a soul mate, a confidant, and a loving and sensitive partner. He levels my sorrow, shares my laughter, sustains me. Together we are stronger, and we drift into sleep so we will be ready for another day.

Daria Davidson: I am a board-certified emergency department physician. Along with another physician, I manage a group of emergency department physicians and provide direct patient care at a Level I Trauma Center/Emergency Department in Wichita, Kansas. I was diagnosed with breast cancer in September 1992, when I was forty-one. I got the results of my biopsy on September 24 and decided on mastectomy and immediate reconstruction, which was performed on September 30. Though only one of my nodes was involved, the type of cancer I had was aggressive, so I opted to enter a clinical trial and bring out the "big guns." My last treatment was on December 31, 1993. I am now back taking care of my patients.

I am told I have a commanding, no-nonsense personality. I am also very organized and enjoy keeping things on track and moving. I and another "straight-ahead" member of this group of contributors acted as coordinators, developing schedules and plans. At first, my openness surprised the others, but luckily when I laughed, everyone else did too; and when I cried, they cried.

For me, Sundays are often just like any other day. I spent this Sunday at the Emergency Department. All seventeen treatment rooms were full and another eight to ten people were waiting to be seen. I had three patients complaining of chest pain, a small child who's having difficulty breathing, two people with minor injuries from an automobile accident, four people complaining of flulike symptoms, another one wanting someone to "stop the voices," a four-month-pregnant woman with unusual bleeding, an elderly patient brought in from the nursing home confused and combative, another person with a possible broken leg, a child with a nosebleed that won't stop, another person complaining of persistent cough (who slips out to smoke a cigarette), and one with stomach cramps that seem to be getting worse. My legs began to hurt only three hours into my twelve-hour shift. I tried hard to be understanding to all the patients, even those who probably didn't need to be here this morning. The stress is unrelenting and comes not from the concerns about the medical problems I'll have to treat, but from not knowing what is wrong with a patient who has to wait while I treat another. Sometimes patients come in faster than I can see them; other times I have to wait on other services for reports before I can move from one patient to the next. We were so busy today, I wasn't sure I would have time to eat. I was lucky to get out of the center by 8:00 P.M. Tonight I have to prepare for Monday's Pediatric Advanced Life Support Instructor's course. I have a little time, though not much, to grab a bite to eat and spend some time with my family. And so it goes, four, five, sometimes six days in a row, with varying shifts. When I have a break of a day or two, there are those phone calls to patients with concerns, chores to do around the house that have gone begging, schedules to prepare, or sleep—precious sleep—to catch up on, to recharge my batteries so that I can start again tomorrow.

Joy Edwards: I have been a real estate broker in Portland, Oregon, for more than twenty-five years. I have been fighting breast cancer for more than nine years—I am a cancer veteran. My first experience with cancer was a diagnosis of early-stage uterine cancer resulting in a hysterectomy. Then in 1984, shortly after having a dream in which I was told I had breast cancer, I discovered a small, elongated mass in my left breast. But because of my husband's critical illness, I put off evaluation until February 1985. After receiving the mammogram results, it was my choice to have the biopsy, and if the results were negative, to have a modified radical mastectomy at the same time. I chose to have the mastectomy. Surgery was followed by chemotherapy and radiation. Two years later, in 1987, I was told that the cancer had metastasized to my spine and lungs. Another round of chemotherapy and radiation followed. During this period, I located in my right breast a mass, which was removed by lumpectomy. I was convinced, at this point, that the breast should be removed, but the doctors did not agree. The treatment seemed to arrest the tumor growth. During this period of treatment, in May 1988, my husband died. In 1990, testing revealed renewed growth, this time in the tumors in both of my lungs. I was treated with chemotherapy. It was during this period of treatment that I discovered another tumor in my breast, and I decided to have a mastectomy of my right breast. In May 1990, I made the decision to discontinue all therapy, to get myself back into condition to deal with the cancer in my lungs. In 1991 surgery was performed on my lungs, and I entered 1992 free of any known cancer activity. By the summer of 1993, I was told I could consider myself to be in remission.

As one of the older members of the group and a veteran of the cancer wars, I felt I needed to show the others that there is hope. I have been through a great deal, and yet I was there, looking normal, being energetic, and ready to be positive and reassuring. I am now working as hard as ever, traveling, and enjoying life.

I doubt that there is such a thing as a normal day in real estate. This day starts at 5:30 with a call from a client who is transferring from Maryland and has forgotten the three-hour time difference. Being already two hours into his day, he was ready to get down to business. I think I will try to get a few additional minutes' sleep, as I spent last evening presenting an offer and didn't get to bed until after midnight. (I decided two years ago that if I worked out of my home, I could take it a little easier. It hasn't really worked out that way.) Phone calls intervene, so I give up and go out to get in a half-hour walk. I vow not to take the mobile phone. Back at my home office, phone calls, scheduling, and rescheduling appointments take up my time until 9:00 A.M., when my assistant arrives to take over the phone. By now, I have already logged over two hours. The rest of the day is spent searching for appropriate homes for new clients, getting properties appraised and reinspected, placing and returning phone calls, and setting up appointments. I pick up a couple who are retiring and want to move from the home in which they have lived for twenty-two years and raised their three children to something smaller. We discuss the marketing strategy for selling their home, a home that holds lifetimes of memories for them. I recognize the need to move slowly, aware that the emotional value these people have invested in their home cannot be discounted; it is not an easy move for them. I make another appointment for 7:00 P.M. to meet some prospective buyers at a piece of property that I think will be well suited to them. I make a quick trip home at about 5:00 P.M. for a bite to eat and a half hour of news before meeting my clients. At 10:40 P.M., my clients see me safely to my car after agreeing on terms.

I finish the day with a call to the listing agent and make arrangements to present the offer tomorrow. Mine is a stressful profession but wonderfully rewarding, and well worth getting up for.

Carol Hebestreit: I am the director of professional relations for Neostrata, Inc., in Princeton, New Jersey. My first experience with cancer was in 1979, when I learned I had malignant melanoma. In 1980, the cancer metastasized to the groin, and I underwent a radical groin dissection. I survived metastatic disease after extensive surgery and BCG (a vaccine that has been tested as a treatment for a number of cancers) therapy—much to the surprise of my health-care team. Then in 1988 I was diagnosed with cancer in my right breast, a second primary tumor. I chose to have a lumpectomy, a partial mastectomy, and node dissection. I did not receive chemotherapy, as my physicians were concerned with a potential compromise of my immune system. I received a full course of radiation and two boosters. To date, my breast cancer has not metastasized.

Having survived the breast cancer experience, as well as malignant melanoma, I am the group's other cancer veteran. I feel that my many years of making decisions regarding my treatments and how they fit in with my demanding profession and single parenthood have helped to give me a perspective that many of the less experienced members of the group have not had time to achieve. I have learned to let go of my fear and anger. I believe I communicated my sense of peace and composure to the other women at the retreat.

Today is, thank God, only somewhat typical. It's 5:00 A.M., and as I head to the shower, I'm wishing I was on my way to exercise rather than to catch a flight to San Francisco from my home in New Jersey for a five-day medical meeting. I get my bags in the car (I decide not to ask Thom for help; he's the love of my life and wonderful, but I don't want to hear about overpacking). Because I have to stop for gas, I arrive at the airport with just ten minutes to collect myself before my boss arrives. I have to conduct an interview in San Francisco while my boss continues on to Monterey, which means I pick up the rental car and drive down the coast of California. I decide there is some justice in the world—the coast is beautiful. However, I lose my way looking for Monterey; it is on the ocean and I instinctively head east for the water. I arrive at the hotel at 4:30 P.M., and I need to have the exhibit set up by 5:00 P.M. and be smiling at three hundred physicians. Only one problem, I've spent twelve hours in these clothes—well, they will just have to do. When I finally get a chance to go to my room for a shower, I discover the suitcase on the bed isn't mine. But in the grand scheme of things, this is nothing to get upset about, and I remain calm. Dinner is great and the company stimulating, though I am fading. I make it back to my room, climb into bed twenty-one hours after leaving home, and find myself thanking God for my wonderful day.

Betsy Lambert: I am an attorney, licensed in several states. I practice in New York City, where I represent both individuals and businesses. On my birthday in 1991, while in Louisiana closing out my law practice there, I discovered a thickening in my breast. After an abnormal mammogram, a sonogram, and two consultations with breast surgeons, I had a biopsy that revealed a one-and-one-quarter-centimeter tumor that was cancerous. I was given the choice of a lumpectomy with radiation or a mastectomy. After several consultations I chose a lumpectomy. A reincision was done two weeks later, to clean the margins and remove the lymph nodes. I had one node involved, which made me a Stage II cancer patient. After the lumpectomy I had six months of chemotherapy and six weeks of radiation. I am not currently taking tamoxifen, although it was recommended.

I am pretty outspoken and at the retreat discovered that I needed to talk about things I hadn't talked about before. When I was with these other women, I was entirely with them, focused and willing to share my most sensitive, private thoughts and feelings. I found it helpful to coordinate and plan schedules; to help keep us to our agenda. And I found out that I could be very funny.

I am up today at 6:30 A.M., thankful that it is not 5:30 A.M. My sleep has changed dramatically because of the premature menopause brought on by the chemotherapy. A good night is one in which I wake up only once or twice. I am amazed I don't seem to suffer from the lack of sleep. I step to the window and take a look at the cityscape. It's a beauty, affording me a view of Lincoln Center and the Hudson River. Because it's snowing, I decide I won't walk through Central Park or exercise but will catch a ride with my husband. Armed with pocketbook/briefcase stuffed with reading material, I arrive at my office at 8:20 A.M., a little late. I check my calendar and the fax machine. Two faxes are waiting for me: a memo from the National Breast Cancer Coalition regarding pending legislation and a contract from one of my corporate clients. The contract needs to be reviewed immediately, as work is to begin in three days. My secretary/assistant arrives at 9:30 and we go over yesterday's work and work priorities for today. I redraft the contract, discuss revisions, fax the redrafts, and amazingly all changes are accepted and the contract finalized. Another client has a crisis. After five calls and some legal research, I give another legal opinion. Two calls later and it's noon.

The mail has arrived, and I receive a judgment on a pending discovery motion in a litigation case. I discuss it with my client, decide on a strategy, draft another motion and a memo to the file. I then check on service of a new complaint, find out it has not been completed, make a notation to my calendar to recheck in two days. A new client arrives for her appointment about a misdiagnosis of breast cancer, and the case looks viable. We discuss the facts of the case, I review hospital records, draft a complaint for the client's approval, and make a call to an expert regarding the case. I get a call from a judge's clerk requesting that a conference among all attorneys be rescheduled. It is hard to say no to a judge. I rush to get to the court on time. I get stopped by the court's metal detector, and my tiny dictating machine is "seized" until I leave. The building is cold, as usual. All counsel file into the judge's chambers, and after clarification of the issues, the attorneys reach some mutual decisions. No one is happy, except the judge, who is finished for the day. I rush out, remembering to pick up my "seized" tape recorder. It's snowing again and I can't find a taxi. I jump on a rush-hour subway and arrive late to a corporate meeting at 6:00 P.M. in Midtown. After the meeting, which lasts until 8:00 P.M., I join my husband and a friend for dinner. We arrive home about 10:30 P.M., just in time to watch the news and relax. I try to get to bed before midnight, and my last thought is, I wonder how I will sleep tonight.

Amy Langer: I have been the executive director of the National Alliance of Breast Cancer Organizations (NABCO) in New York City since 1990. I was thirty years old when I was diagnosed, almost ten years ago. In the course of a routine checkup, my gynecologist casually suggested that I get a mammogram. That mammogram proved suspicious. After a few months of waiting and watching under the care of a surgeon, I was given the diagnosis of early-stage invasive breast cancer. I elected to have a lumpectomy. There was no node involvement. I underwent eight weeks of daily radiation therapy.

Because of preexisting commitments and travel plans, I was not able to attend the retreat, but I have been in frequent contact with my cocontributors and members of the IMEC staff.

Today, I am up by 7:30 A.M. and spend the next hour and a half preparing for the day, with my baby playing around my feet. I get to my office at 9:15 and grab a quick breakfast at my desk. My computer and phone are like appendages, I spend so much time with them. I schedule two public speaking engagements for next week. After returning several phone calls, I meet with some of the members of my staff to review the status of a number of projects in progress. Today, like most days, I eat my lunch at my desk. After lunch, which consisted of cookies and a piece of fruit, I head across town to meet with a pharmaceutical company that has requested information on appropriate marketing approaches for a product they are introducing for breast cancer patients. There are a ton of faxes to read when I get back to my office, including a speech to review and approve that Paula Zahn will be giving at our annual luncheon next week. There are also faxes from a federal agency regarding an issue involving the FDA. I have several interviews for staff positions scheduled for this afternoon. After returning several more phone calls, but before my first interview, I review the Alliance's operating budget. The interviews are interesting; some very qualified people have applied. I spend the last hour before going home working on requests for information on clinical trial recruitment and on confirming my schedule for tomorrow. Today I make it out of the office by 5:00 P.M. and head home to spend the time till 8:00 P.M. with my son.

Cathy Masamitsu: I am a television producer in Los Angeles; one of the shows I am involved with is *The Home Show.* I have faced two diagnoses of breast cancer, the first when I was thirty-two. After the first diagnosis, I had a lumpectomy and six weeks of radiation therapy, followed by an implanted iridium "boost." A recurrence of the cancer was detected in 1989—I was thirty-five. I chose to undergo a modified radical mastectomy and immediate reconstruction. I received neither chemotherapy nor hormonal therapy for either occurrence. The support and strength I receive from my mother and family and my deep Christian faith are, in great measure, responsible for my triumph over breast cancer each time I have faced this disease.

Some of the other contributors already "knew" me from the programs we have aired on *The Home Show* about my experiences with breast cancer. I feel a responsibility as a member of the media to make an effort to broadcast empowering information about breast health, and I believe that it is important for all of us to look at broader issues for women living with breast cancer.

It's 5:15 A.M. and still dark. I leave my house dressed in jeans, sweatshirt, and sneakers, with my on-camera wardrobe draped over one arm. I close the front door with care, so I don't wake Mom or my brother David, saying my prayers in the car as the sun rises. Television is exciting work, but *live* television—now that's really exciting. There aren't too many shows aired live anymore. I am going in early because I'm on the show today. I've been working for ten days on the segment we are airing today and only got back a few days ago from London, where I traveled to report on the story. I'll be talking about an innovative chemotherapy study published recently by the Royal Marsden Cancer Hospital. I am so fortunate to have a job I love, and one that *helps people*. I arrive at the studio, which is busy with activity. I check the fax machine, retrieving information from the Marsden that I will use today. Everything is last minute on this job; I always think I'll get used to it, but I never do. I report to the hair and makeup room early for my 6:00 A.M. call time and hand the fax to one of the producers, requesting the script be altered to include the new information. We walk through the segment as I am being "miked." It's almost 8:00 A.M.—show time! These few minutes before show time are filled with nervous tension. I love the feeling—so alive—it's electrifying. The show's over. The segment is a hit. I walk upstairs to my office and the other part of my job, that of assistant to Executive Producer Woody Fraser, a role I have filled for over thirteen years. I attack the huge pile of phone messages as the phone begins to ring. I juggle production schedules for three different shows currently in production. I am a good troubleshooter and I hope I have left everyone with the feeling that they are number one. I gratefully accept a coworker's offer to bring me something for lunch from the commissary. I quickly eat my lunch at my desk, trying to catch up on my never-ending pile of reading material, both business and personal. Woody's day usually ends early, but mine never does. I spend the afternoon arranging my calendar to include a couple of speeches for the American Cancer Society in Chicago and Atlanta next month. A colleague calls to tell me about a friend who was diagnosed today with breast cancer; I put together a packet of resource materials for her, barely getting it downstairs in time for the FedEx pickup. I fax Woody a revision to tomorrow's agenda. Finally, at 6:30 P.M., I leave for a Deacon Board meeting at my church, which lasts till 10:00. It is almost as dark when I head home as it was when I left, and I end the day as I began it, with a prayer of thanksgiving.

Sally Snodgrass: I am a Ph.D. and social psychologist at Florida Atlantic University. I was diagnosed with breast cancer (no node involvement) in 1990 at age forty-seven. I elected to have a lumpectomy followed by radiation. Following a bout with unidentified, intermittent back pain, it was discovered that the cancer had metastasized to the lymph nodes in my lower abdomen. I was given a course of tamoxifen, which failed to help. I began chemotherapy in November 1991, which continued throughout 1992. Chemotherapy was discontinued, as the nodes remained stable. When the pain increased, I began treatment with a stronger chemotherapy. In August 1993, I underwent a stem-cell transplant and am recovering.

Because I was still in the hospital, in protective isolation, recovering from the stem-cell transplant, I was unable to attend the retreat in person. I did, however, participate via speakerphone. Though I was able to participate in only a few of the sessions, I felt a real connection with the group. It was a wonderful sharing experience, and I think we all learned from each other.

I wake up at 6:30 and my first thought is of coffee—coffee is what gets me out of bed. I sip my coffee and set up my VCR for twenty minutes of exercise. Then, after ten minutes of prayer and meditation, I am ready to dress, make lunch, plan my day. I drive the five minutes to the Social Sciences Building. The south Florida weather, as usual, is beautiful—sunny and warm with a constant sea breeze. I would love to go to the beach, but I do not. I chat with the secretary and other faculty before going to my office and tackling the business of the day. My desk is buried in stacks of journals, junk mail, old exams, research projects in progress, and lecture notes. Someday, I *must* get organized. But right now I need to concentrate on today's lectures. I remember to look for a better example of stereotyping—the one I used last time didn't go over well. I feel satisfied that I am prepared, at least for today. I look over the course schedules for the next few weeks and order the film I want for a discussion on aggression. I spend some time with a student trying to find ways for him to better study and prepare for class. Lunch is the sandwich I made this morning. I head to the lecture hall. Class sizes are way too large! When will we learn to invest enough money in education? Once I begin, I get into my "altered state of teaching," in which I become oblivious to time passing. It is so much easier now than it was those first few years out of graduate school. The lectures go well. I really enjoy these classes—and the challenge of keeping a hundred-plus students attentive and interested. I am back in my office and exhausted. Even after eleven years of doing this, it is still a strain. How do other professors make it look so easy? But then, maybe it *looks* easy when I do it, too. I spend the rest of the afternoon in committee meetings, preparing for my seminar tomorrow night, setting up my research project on sex differences in assuming leadership. Jim (my significant other) calls and we plan dinner tonight. After dinner, we must get those reservations made for the ski trip to Colorado over Christmas break! Time is running out . . .

Carol Stack: I am a Ph.D. in anthropology and a professor of women's studies and education at the University of California, Berkeley. I was diagnosed with breast cancer in March 1993. A month later I had a lumpectomy. I was node negative, had not yet gone a full year without having a period, and my tumor was found to be estrogen positive. I received a six-month course of chemotherapy (CMF) and seven weeks of radiation. I am currently debating whether or not to take tamoxifen. I am the "youngest" of the contributors in terms of length of time since diagnosis and was in the midst of therapy during the retreat and the writing of the book.

I steered our conversations to issues of work and money and social class, often drawing the comparison between our situation as professional and working women to women without jobs or health benefits. I am generally soft-spoken but very committed to issues of race, class, and social policy. Some of my co-contributors said I reminded them of the 1960s when commitment to social reform was more a part of our social conscience than it is today.

Exercise only happens in my life early in the morning. I meet my friend Jill at 6:30 A.M. and we walk up a steep road and back—four miles round-trip. The walk gets my joints lubricated and makes it easier to go home and sit in front of my computer for a couple of hours to work on my book. I claim to be a night person, but mornings are reserved for doing research at home. By 11:00 A.M. I am on campus for a women's studies meeting. I finish preparing for class at a café off campus and realize that I am late. I run across the entire campus to give my lecture titled Race, Gender, and Class. I spend the rest of the afternoon reading and preparing to meet with my research team. Dinner doesn't happen. But I did put two apples in my backpack this morning. I meet with the team at 6:30 P.M. to go over what they have learned about the meaning of work for youth in the labor force. All of the research assistants are working at fast-food restaurants to get hands-on information and insight. I get home about 9:00

P.M. I see I have ten messages on my answering machine. One caller asked me to be an expert witness in a child custody case, another to discuss a meeting to consider strategies for implementing a pay equity study. I settle down to read an armful of essays and review proposals for senior thesis projects. I finally put aside the essays and proposals and dig into a great novel, *Mad Blood,* by David Nemec. I turn the light out about midnight.

Carol Washington: I have been the community relations coordinator for Cancer Care, Inc., in New York City since 1968. In 1991 a routine mammogram revealed a spot that warranted additional exploration. A biopsy was performed. The results showed a one-centimeter infiltrating ductal carcinoma in my left breast. I had breast cancer. My lumpectomy was followed two months later with a regimen of radiation treatments. At age fifty-seven, I had become one of "those" statistics.

Maybe being the oldest in the group accounts for why I was the only one who did not cry openly during the retreat. Each experience shared by the others penetrated me deeply. It wasn't easy remaining dry-eyed. Perhaps, too, it was instinct that made me feel that I needed to provide a steadying force (learned behavior) and share the strength that I derive daily from my abiding faith and belief in God and my love for others.

It's 5:45 A.M. and my internal alarm has beaten the clock again. Another small victory. I am brushing my teeth when I realize that someone is talking to my answering machine. I dash but am too late. So what else is new, it's Thursday. Energized now and moving faster, I pop my tamoxifen pill, reach for the phone to return the earlier call, then stop. How can I start my day without a prayer? This day must be acknowledged and embraced with thanksgiving and praise. I'm alive and able to add another twenty-four hours to the distance from that unpleasant moment of diagnosis. Later I begin to mentally review my agenda for the day and wonder how many things I will have checked off by the end of the day. My two-minute walk to the subway turns into a sprint when I hear the train coming. I choose to use this morning's ride to review my class research paper rather than just gaze out the window. (I'm enrolled in a graduate program with classes in the evenings.) I become so engrossed in my reading that I miss my stop, and what should be a forty-five-minute ride turns into a seventy-five-minute odyssey and an extra walk. Once in my office, a day's activities begin, starting with one or two attempts at downing a hot cup of tea (poor success rate), returning phone calls, proofreading newsletter copy, rearranging an appointment that took forever to set up, and talking shop with people while walking from one area to another (normal activity). An early doctor's appointment enables me to enjoy a brisk one-mile walk, round-trip, from the subway to the hospital. Back in the office, copy is drafted for guest presenters participating in a special agency event; the conversation ebbs and flows with the event's master of ceremonies, a printer, and other staff (in public relations, communication with others is a constant activity). A glance at my watch tells me it's 2:30 P.M., causing me to wonder what will assuage my hunger until I get home, which will be around 9:30 P.M., since I have a class tonight. Two juicy sausages with mustard and sauerkraut from the man on the corner would be divine. And this day is only half over.

Summary of Medical Events for Contributors

Authors	D.C.	D.D.	J.E.	C.H.
Initial Diagnosis				
Detection method	BSE	BSE	BSE	BSE
Date of primary diagnosis	8/90	9/92	2/85	11/88
Date of biopsy	8/90	9/92	2/85	11/88
Date of surgery	9/90 (L)	9/92 (M)	2/85 (M)	11/88 (L, partial M)
Reconstruction	N	Y	N	N
Stage at primary diagnosis	II	II	II	I
Chemotherapy	Y	Y	Y	N
Radiation	Y	N	Y	Y
Radiation boosts	Y	N	N	Y
Hormone therapy	N; Y (R)	N	Y	N
Recurrence/Metastasis				
Date of recurrence/ metastasis	93 (ME)	N	87 (ME) 88 (R) 90 (ME) 91 (ME) (R)	N
Date of surgery	N	N	87 (L) 88 (M) 91 (PN)	N
Reconstruction	N	N	N	N
Chemotherapy	Y	N	Y	N
Radiation	Y	N	Y	N
Stem-cell transplant	5/94	N	N	N

Code: BSE = breast self-exam; Mam = mammography;
L = lumpectomy; M = mastectomy; PN = pneumonectomy;
R = recurrence; ME = metastasis; N = no/none; Y= yes

B.L.	A.L.	C.M.	S.S.	C.S.	C.W.
BSE	Mam	BSE	BSE	BSE	Mam
5/91	10/84	3/86	9/90	2/93	5/91
5/91	10/84	4/86	9/90	2/93	6/91
6/91 (L)	11/84 (L)	4/86 (L)	9/90 (L)	3/93 (L)	6/91 (L)
N	N	N	N	N	N
II	I	0	I	II	II
Y	N	N	N	Y	N
Y	Y	Y	Y	Y	Y
N	Y	Y	N	Y	Y
N	N	N	Y	N	Y
N	N	89 (R)	91 (ME)	N	N
N	N	89 (M)	N	N	N
N	N	Y	N	N	N
N	N	N	Y	N	N
N	N	N	N	N	N
N	N	N	8/93	N	N

Facts About Breast Cancer

- Statistically, one out of nine women in the United States will develop breast cancer in her lifetime—a risk that was one out of fourteen in 1960. This year, a woman will be newly diagnosed with breast cancer every three minutes, and a woman will die from breast cancer every twelve minutes.
- Breast cancer is the most common form of cancer in women in the United States. Both its cause and the means for its cure remain undiscovered. About two million breast cancer survivors are alive in America today.
- In 1997, 180,200 new cases of female invasive breast cancer will be diagnosed, and 43,900 women will die from the disease.
- Breast cancer is the second leading cause of cancer death for all women and the leading cause of death in women between the ages of forty and fifty-five.
- Every woman is at risk for breast cancer. Seventy percent of women diagnosed with breast cancer have no identifiable risk factors.
- Women who have inadequate access to quality medical care die from breast cancer at a higher rate

than other women, a direct result of diagnosis at later stages.

- Accurate, up-to-date information can decrease anxiety, increase self-esteem, facilitate decisionmaking, and improve overall recovery and adjustment.
- Many breast lumps are found by women themselves, yet few women practice breast self-examination (BSE) regularly and often don't know how to do so properly.
- Breast cancer cannot be prevented. Early detection offers the best chance to treat the disease successfully, yet fewer than half of American women aged forty and older have regular screening mammograms. The National Cancer Institute now recommends screening mammograms every one to two years for women beginning at age forty.

Breast Cancer?
Let Me Check My Schedule!

1

The Shock of Diagnosis

"At the time, the most horrendous thing I could imagine was someone sticking a needle in my breast."
—*Cathy Masamitsu*

For as long as we can remember, we have taken charge of our lives. We set goals and don't give up until they are reached. We have worked hard to establish ourselves personally and professionally and have learned our lessons on the way up. We plan, organize, prioritize, set goals, and draw up schedules rather than risk leaving events to outside influences. We are accustomed to structuring our own lives and making our own decisions, and to being rewarded with success. We accept more responsibilities and duties than do our peers. We have earned a reputation for being dependable and "exceptionally competent." Others rely on us.

Control is a fundamental part of our natures. To us, control means discipline, freedom, self-determination, independence, self-reliance, and choice. It is a key element of our outlook on life and an essential underpinning of our success.

The feeling of being in control deserted us in an instant when we received our diagnoses of breast cancer. We were not prepared for it, and our reactions ranged from confusion and despair to panic:

> "It was like there was an exam and I wasn't ready."
> "Suddenly I was on a playing field and I didn't know the game."
> "I felt like I was in a foreign country and hadn't studied the language."
> "Suddenly other people were controlling my destiny and I felt ignorant."
> "I wasn't used to feeling unprepared—to feeling out of my depth."

This is how it happened for us.

≶≷

Carol W. I never worried about cancer. High blood pressure, hypertension, and stroke were the diseases that struck my family on my mother's side. Old age, for the most part, was the cause on my father's side. I always felt that if anything happened to me, it would be one of those diseases African-Americans seem prone to, but certainly not cancer. It is not "our" disease. I work for Cancer Care, Inc., which affords me access to a great deal of useful material. Articles on the subject cross our desks with regularity, and I am an agency spokesperson on the services we provide. I knew something about cancer but I always thought "All this applies to other people, not to me."

Having let two years go by without one, I had a mammogram in May 1991. The doctor who interpreted the film tried to make light of a suspicious spot, telling me that most of these lumps turn out to be benign. She suggested further examination by my own doctor, which I agreed to. Being a somewhat private and very self-controlled person, I went back to my office and didn't say anything to anyone except one social worker friend. She gave me a new directory to scan that had recently been compiled by one of our volunteers. One doctor's name kept showing up as a good doctor and a good person to talk to, and she was part of our health-care plan. I made an appointment, which had to be changed twice.

I said nothing to my daughter or anyone else in my family. Being used to the role of family care provider, the person who ran the show, I didn't want to convey anything that would make me appear vulnerable or weak. It wasn't my style. Besides, I hadn't acknowledged that something might be wrong. My usual schedule kept me busy—working, taking classes in the evening, fulfilling my volunteer obligations, being active in church. There was enough to keep me occupied. But in the quiet of night, I kept studying the mammogram, trying to unravel the significance of the little spot on the film.

The day of my appointment with the new doctor arrived. She looked at the film and recommended a biopsy, which could be done on an outpatient basis. We talked about the procedure and arranged for the surgery, then I went back to work. I'm always going back to the office! Now it was time to share what was occurring, just in case. Two of my colleagues had that dubious honor, and they were wonderful. Thus began a process of accepting caring arms around me.

My biopsy was really a lumpectomy with the whole lump and immediate surrounding area removed. My doctor saw no need to do two procedures when one would suffice. She asked me to call her the next day to discuss the pathology report. I felt within myself that "this is not good, I don't like this at all." In retrospect, I was scared. When I called, she suggested that I come to her office the next day for a conference. I told her I couldn't come because Friday was the annual Fund-Raising Executives of New York event, and it was important for me to be there. She told me she needed to see me.

At lunchtime I left the Waldorf Astoria Hotel and took a cab to the doctor's office. "I have bad news for you. The tumor was malignant, very small, one centimeter, and we're lucky to have caught it so early." She discussed therapeutic options for me to consider and encouraged me to seek a second and third opinion if I wanted to do so. No decision was necessary immediately.

This woman made me feel so very, very special. I wondered if she'd had breast cancer herself. To this day I don't know, but that was the kind of empathy she conveyed—"I know exactly what you are going through." After assuring her that I was okay to travel alone, I walked to the subway, waited patiently for my train, and took a nap (a normal thing for me), and didn't deal with the diagnosis. I couldn't accept the news. I denied it. Too many sad and painful things had been happening in my life in a relatively short period of time. Death seemed to be all around me. Within the last couple of years, my mother had died after a long, debilitating illness; two extremely close, sisterlike friends passed away; and several other people who had been special were gone. It wasn't an easy time. But I am a strong person and I would handle this situation myself, relying on me, as usual.

I received the diagnosis on a Friday afternoon and spent the weekend at home by myself. I didn't answer the telephone, my answering machine was full. On Sunday I went to church—part of my denial—after all, I had responsibilities, a Sunday school class to teach. At the end of the day, one of my "sisters" (I have no biological ones) called me over and asked what was bothering me, noticing that I didn't seem to be myself. I caved in and told her. It was my first release. This great rock of Gibraltar finally broke. I cried and cried and was just a total wreck. She cried too, and we couldn't do anything for what seemed like an eternity. After years of being the provider/caregiver, being strong, being the shoulder to cry on, being the one who always held up, I was able to let myself go and be human. Superwoman disappeared for a few hours.

᭚᭚

Carol S. During the last week of February 1993, I was a guest speaker for a conference at Dartmouth. I gave a lecture from my new book on African-Americans returning home to rural southern communities. It was a wonderful occasion and terribly exciting, since we were celebrating the tenth anniversary of the Rockefeller Center for Social Sciences at Dartmouth. I was scheduled to fly back to California early the next morning. That night the last big snow of the winter fell, and no one could go anywhere. I hadn't carried tremendous files of work with me, and so I had absolute time to myself. For once I had a day that wasn't crammed from seven in the morning to late at night with classes to teach, meetings with students and colleagues, and other things I had to do. I took a long walk in the snow, enjoying every moment. That evening I was lying in bed and I decided it was a perfect time to do a really thorough breast check. I felt quite sensual and happy. I was proud of myself for doing a breast self-exam and I was very thorough.

Near the surface of my right breast, on the outside, I noticed something that felt like a raisin, about that size and that soft. I experimented a little bit, thinking, I wonder if I could find it again? and each time I did find the lump, but I didn't take it seriously. I finally said, "Hell, I'll just go to sleep. It'll be gone in the morning." It seemed almost like a dream sequence with the snow piled up outside and being in this lovely room in a bed-and-breakfast.

The next morning I checked my breast and the lump was still there. It was a real surprise to me. I called my gynecologist in Berkeley and said, "I think I'd better see you on Monday." We set that up and I flew home.

My gynecologist said it looked suspicious. When I raised my arm, she could see a bit of a dent. She knew a surgeon and arranged for me to see him right away for a biopsy. Still I was totally convinced that it wouldn't be cancer. I knew that only 10 percent of biopsies turn out to be malignant, and at that time there was no history of cancer in my family. I had all these lively, elderly aunts who'd lived a long time. I didn't know much about breast cancer or any other disease because I'd never been interested in medicine. I'd always assumed if anything was going to get me it would be emphysema, since that's what got my father. I was sure that I didn't have breast cancer. I was really sure. When the doctor told me it was malignant, I was shocked. I was incredulous. I didn't believe it. Ten percent took on a totally new meaning to me. Still I was stoic. Months later, I'm not sure the diagnosis—the fact that I have breast cancer—has really hit me yet.

When I think back to how I "remember" my reaction to the diagnosis, I realize that I had created "my cancer story." For months before and even after our retreat, I had consistently told people the same story about finding the lump during my trip to Dartmouth. Each of us works out a shorthand for presenting ourselves and for explaining our predicament, especially, when in the surprise of illness we find ourselves asked to tell, over and over again to caring friends and workmates, how we found our lump. It wasn't until I had time to examine my "story" that I realized what I had left out. Maybe I only acknowledged the possibility of a lump while I was staying in an inn far from home. Who knows? I do know that over the many months of conversation after I was diagnosed, I never once mentioned that my partner had noticed a hardness in my breast the month preceding the trip to Dartmouth. He had worried about it, reminded me of it, and urged me several times to have it checked. That was the impetus for my self-exam; it was the shock of the diagnosis that wiped that part of the story from my spoken memory.

Sally. I found a lump in July 1990 when I scratched an itch on my breast in the middle of the night. My January mammogram had not shown any problems. I have pretty lumpy breasts, anyway, so I did not panic then. I waited until after my period to see if it was still there. Two years earlier, my mother had died of breast cancer. I thought my demise would probably be breast cancer, too, but not now. Mother was sixty-eight. I was only forty-seven. After my period the lump was still there, so I went to my internist. After an ultrasound, he sent me to a surgeon, who wanted to do a biopsy. I had things planned. My life was too full to take time out right then for surgery. I asked if it would be risky to wait until after a professional meeting, a visit with friends in New York, and a scuba diving trip planned for Labor Day weekend. The doctor was surprised. He said, "Most women are in a big hurry to find out. But I don't think a month is going to make a difference." So I did what I planned to do and then scheduled my biopsy.

When I heard the diagnosis (over the telephone), I was shocked. I had assumed that this was a benign lump like so many that had been removed from women on my mother's side of the family. Cancer at forty-seven? Mom died after a miserable fight with both chemotherapy and radiation. Is that all I had left? Throwing up and getting weak and then dying? I haven't even found my "life's purpose" yet. What have I done for the world? What have I experienced? I'm not anywhere near finished!

I had a lumpectomy with an axillary dissection and radiation. It was a tiny lump, and my lymph nodes were negative. We all thought I was in the category of 95 percent cure rate without the need for chemotherapy. This experience was just a "notice" to begin accomplishing whatever I wanted to accomplish. Thank you, God, for the "kick in the pants."

I was experiencing intermittent lower back pain in the fall of 1990 and spring of 1991. I went to my internist and to a chiropractor and told them I was in pain, but they wouldn't listen. It was just "muscle strain." I had X rays and tests. Finally, the doctor suggested that it was stress and I needed to see a psychotherapist. If I had followed his advice, I would be dead now. Instead, I remembered a CT scan (often called a CAT scan) from September 1990 that had something questionable on it that everyone ignored. I pulled that out and took it to the internist and asked, "Could this have anything to do with my back pain?" We did another CT scan, which showed greatly enlarged lymph nodes in the lower abdomen, and I was sent to an oncologist immediately. My breast cancer had metastasized to the lymph system in my lower back area. This diagnosis was the hardest of all. I read the statistics. Only 15 percent of metastasized breast cancer patients lived five years. This was so unfair. I was so young. I was so unfinished.

⋙⋘

Cathy. I was thirty-two years old the first time I was diagnosed with breast cancer. That was eight years ago. I'd never had a mammogram, since I was so young, but luckily my mother had taught me to check my breasts and raised me with the belief that I needed to be aware of my body and of any changes. Late on Friday night, I was checking my breasts and I found a lump. It wasn't hard. It was rubbery and square and flat. I woke up my mom— she lives with me—and she said, "It's probably nothing, honey. I get those fatty tumors all the time, but you should have it checked on Monday." I don't think I worried at first about the lump being cancer. I worried that I didn't know what it was and didn't even know anything about what a mammogram entailed. My ignorance about the procedures added to my anxiety. I did a lot of praying that weekend.

I called my family doctor at eight-thirty Monday morning and caught him just as he got to his office. He told me to come right over and he'd examine me, then refer me for a mammogram. I had my first mammogram and it looked fine, but since my breast tissue was so dense, they sent me with my films to meet with a surgeon. This was unexpected and made me really nervous. "Why do I need a surgeon?" I asked myself as I drove the few blocks to the other office. The surgeon turned out to be a wonderful man, very warm and easy to talk to, a "hugging" person with a broad smile. I liked him right from the start. He explained to me that he would be giving me a needle aspiration, and even apologized for the fact that it might hurt a little bit. He reassured me that it was "probably nothing," and a few days later the results came back benign. I was so relieved at first and then somewhat stunned when he added, "I still think we should remove it if it isn't gone in a month or so." A month later the lump was still there, so I scheduled an outpatient biopsy surgery. The doctor explained, "I'm not worried about it, but there's no reason to leave it in there. We won't know what it is for sure until we take it out." I was astonished that they had no way to determine what the lump was without cutting me. I wasn't worried about cancer, but I didn't want a scar on my breast, and I spent some tearful nights before the day of surgery.

They gave me a local anesthetic and began to remove the lump. My family doctor was there with the surgeon, which made me feel as safe and comfortable as you can be in such a situation. As the surgeon removed the lump, he said, "Oh, here it comes . . . it's a boy! What do you want to name him?" I asked what the lump looked like, and the surgeon said, "Like a piece of fat you'd cut off a steak." They didn't think the lump was anything serious. They carried the lump of fat over to the lab, and the moment the pathologist cut through it, they could see the cancer.

My doctors told me right then that it looked like a malignancy. My surgeon was disappointed and upset. He said to my doctor, "Goddammit, Bob, they have to do something about mammograms. They're not reliable enough. I've seen too many young women like Cathy who find out like this. This is not right . . ." My doctors were having a heated discussion about how it wasn't fair and I was thinking, I have cancer? What does this mean?

They closed me up and told me I'd have to spend the night in the hospital so they could do a lumpectomy the next day. I thought, Wait a minute. I wasn't expecting this. I just took the afternoon off and now . . . Then I thought of my mother and realized that outside the operating room someone was telling her that her daughter had breast cancer. I felt overwhelmingly helpless.

I pictured my mother out in the hall or somewhere else in the hospital hearing the news and I felt terrible. I wanted to tell her myself. I didn't know who was telling her or how. That was very hard for me. I'm a person who lives and feels a lot through the people closest to me. When I look back, I think maybe part of my concern for my family was a result of my not knowing how to deal with my own reaction to the diagnosis. But the overwhelming concern I felt at that moment was for my family and what my diagnosis would mean to them.

To my mother, it would mean I was going to die. I knew that. As a Christian, I've never been afraid of death, so I wasn't terribly concerned about whether or not my diagnosis meant I was going to die. But I knew that even just the doctor's announcement that I had to stay in the hospital that night would say to my mother that there was a great chance she was going to lose me.

Amy. Ten years ago I was a senior vice president in corporate finance at a Wall Street investment bank. Those were the times when young people worked ninety hours a week, had high levels of power and responsibility, and earned alarming amounts of money. I was thirty years old. Although my mother had died from cancer, it was not breast cancer, so I knew very little about it. The thought had never occurred to me that I was at risk. During a routine checkup, my gynecologist furrowed his brow and said to me, "You know, you are so lumpy that it's hard to examine you. Understand, your breasts feel perfectly normal, but why don't you go ahead and get a mammogram." I got dressed, added this item to my Filofax under "medium level priority," item number eleven, and went back to work.

About a month later, I made an appointment for a mammogram the following month. I was annoyed when I glanced at my calendar and saw the appointment for the next afternoon, since I was in the middle of a securities offering and really pressed for time. Grumbling, I went anyway, taking along a legal tote bursting with documents and highlighters in several colors. I had the mammogram and was back in the waiting room, my papers spread out on the floor and across four chairs, when the technician appeared at the door, cocking a finger at me. "Could you come back in, please? There's something we need to take another look at." Next they were drawing on my left breast with a ballpoint pen. I spent the next few months waiting and watching under the care of a surgeon, confident that it was nothing. That nothing turned out to be early-stage invasive breast cancer.

The events that unfolded after that could come from anyone's story. Disbelief, fear, panic. A hundred phone calls, a second opinion, the tour of radiation oncologist's and plastic surgeon's offices. Tears, alone at night, since I was recently separated from my husband. A stiff upper lip at the office, where I explained the situation briefly and then buried myself in work. Finally, a pivotal discussion with a friend in Europe who told me that mastectomies were becoming passé. I shopped until I found a breast surgeon who would perform a lumpectomy and had it done. I went back to work the next week. Thank goodness, no nodes were involved. Daily radiation therapy for eight weeks would be no big deal. Life could go on—this was just a blip, a brief interruption.

Except life doesn't just go on. No matter into which far corner of the brain you try to push it, having a diagnosis of breast cancer changes everything. I was not superwoman, in control of all the details, after all.

⨳

Betsy. Breast cancer was not something I ever thought about. I was amazingly healthy. I'd never had any medical problems. I didn't understand the medical system, didn't understand hospitals, and didn't understand doctors. I'd only gone to the hospital to have my two daughters. That was the extent of my involvement with the medical system. And that was fine with me.

I had my first mammogram at forty-four—nothing, clean, everything's fine. Great. Three years later, in March, I was reading a book, and when I flung my hand out something felt different—there was a lump, a hard place in my breast, right under the muscle. I assumed I'd bruised myself, but I couldn't remember bumping into anything or hurting myself in any way. I thought, "Ah, that's really weird. Maybe I should go see about this. Maybe I should go have a mammogram."

My gynecologist was out of town, but I screamed and carried on until the technician gave me a mammogram. It was fine. Nothing. But I felt I needed to do something, even though I didn't want to. I thought that nagging feeling must be a symptom of menopause. I told myself, "You've got a clean mammogram. You're fine. It couldn't be anything." I didn't think for a second, not for a second, that I might have breast cancer. At the urging of my family, I called to make an appointment with a breast surgeon who is well known in New York City. The receptionist said, "Oh, you have a negative mammogram, ma'am, it will be three months before the doctor can see you." On the day of my appointment, I sat in the waiting room for four hours before the surgeon could see me. I felt four hours was a bit too long to wait to talk to a physician. I wanted someone who was much more personal. So I went to Memorial Sloan-Kettering Cancer

Center and insisted upon having a woman surgeon, and she suggested a biopsy.

I was concerned that she might get me into surgery and decide the lump was malignant and do a mastectomy right then and there. She said, "No, I'd never do that. It will be a biopsy only." I wasn't particularly intimidated. I still didn't think for a second that I might have breast cancer. I thought, Well, I'll go for the biopsy, no big deal.

Later, all the women who'd had biopsies that day were lined up in little chairs down the hall. I saw my doctor coming. She passed the first woman, no problem, passed the next one, and kept on coming, down, down, down the hall until she got to me. She stopped in front of me and said, "May I see you in the room across the hall?" I thought, "That's it, boom, it's me." When she told me it was cancer, I didn't hear anything else. I didn't hear anything else for the rest of the day. Absolutely nothing. I don't think I heard anything for about a week.

I was terrified. My father died six months after he was diagnosed with cancer, so I thought, "That's it! I'm dead!" I was totally devastated. I was afraid I was going to scream or lose control, and that would be unfair to the people around me. I needed to keep some type of control. I left the hospital. I went outside and I walked and walked and walked. I was so overwhelmed by the diagnosis, so emotionally unprepared for it. I was forty-eight at the time, and you'd think that somebody that age would have thought about death and dying in a little bit more detail than I had, but it was almost as if it had never occurred to me that someday I'd have to die. Except for my father, everybody in my family lived such long lives that I just assumed you died in your eighties and you didn't die from any disease but simply went to sleep in a chair and didn't wake up. That's the way I thought people died. Except for my father. He was the only person in my family who had died from an illness. And it was cancer. And it was quick.

I thought, "I'm dead. Yeah, I'll probably have the surgery and the chemo, but I'll be dead in six months. I better write my will and say 'I'm sorry' to all those people who I should have apologized to a long time ago. I'd better make a list of people to say good-bye to." That's exactly what I thought. I didn't think I'd be alive in two years. I thought once you have the diagnosis of cancer, you just automatically die, no matter what the medical establishment said. As far as I was concerned, I might not even make it through surgery. I had, of course, been to law school and read all those cases about people who went into the hospital with an ingrown toenail and lost their lives. I'd be one of those statistics up on the wall, one of those pathetic cases in a textbook.

Nothing in life meant anything. It was a good three days before I could pull myself together. First I had to bury myself and say good-bye to a bunch of people. I had to make amends. I had to call an old boyfriend and tell him I was sorry I'd dropped him back in the 1960s. I started calling people. My friends would say, "What are you doing? What's happening that you're saying good-bye to us?" And a few of them said, "Maybe you should think about this a little bit more. You're clearly deranged right now." Thank goodness I called only my good friends.

⇔

Carol H. The first and second times I was diagnosed with cancer, I felt fear; the third time I felt anger. In 1979, I was diagnosed with malignant melanoma. The surgeons removed the tumors, did a skin graft, and told me I was fine and not to worry another thing about it. A year later

I received a promotion and moved with my two young sons from Ft. Lauderdale to corporate headquarters in New Jersey. Soon after, I was applying body cream following my bath and discovered a lump in my left groin. I thought, Who in the world can help me find a physician? I didn't know a soul in New Jersey, and I was practically the only professional woman at my company. Eventually, I found a warm, gentle man at work who gave me the name of a physician in New Jersey. My appointment was on a Friday. On the following Monday, they operated and discovered the melanoma had metastasized. I was sent to Memorial Sloan-Kettering in New York City for a radical groin dissection and BCG therapy.

Eight years later, at the age of forty-one, in 1988, I was smoothing lotion on my skin and I found a lump in my breast. Being a patient at Sloan-Kettering, I'd had mammograms regularly, and my baseline was fine. No family history of breast cancer. As soon as I found the lump, I had a mammogram; it looked fine, although there were a few calcifications, and my physicians weren't concerned. They asked me to wait for a couple of menses, thinking that some change might show up then. But the lump felt unusual and different, and the situation made me uneasy. I returned to Sloan-Kettering for a needle biopsy followed by a lumpectomy. The diagnosis was medullary carcinoma. My significant other, Thom, was with me when I heard the news. He cried when he heard. My reaction was unbridled anger!

I was already furious with the medical system, outraged at the way women were treated. I was devastated by the loss of my thirty-five-year-old sister, who had died of AIDS just nine months before. I'd spent two years fighting the medical establishment on her behalf. She had experienced chronic colds, fatigue, and skin rashes, and none of the numerous medical experts she consulted were able to determine what was wrong. Finally, a dermatologist did a blood test, and Kathy was diagnosed HIV-positive. In 1986, a six-foot-tall, beautiful heterosexual woman couldn't possibly be HIV-positive according to the medical experts. She was denied experimental drugs because she didn't fit the criteria. When she was finally given the drugs, it was too late. She fought a courageous battle and two years later, weighing just eighty-two pounds, died of AIDS.

When they told me the tumor in my breast was malignant, I wasn't sure I wanted to take care of it. I'd just watched my sister endure treatment that wasn't even humane. I didn't want physicians to deny my femininity and cut my breast off or whatever they chose to do. Right after my diagnosis, I rebelled and denied the tumor. Then I reached a decision point: Did I want to live? Did I want to go through treatment for breast cancer? I sought out a number of women who were survivors of breast cancer and tried to talk through my feelings. I avoided the medical community because I didn't think doctors would help me. I needed other women who had already experienced what I would have to go through. These women helped me deal with my own diagnosis. Eventually, I came around in a way that I never thought I would. These courageous women brought me to a stage of believing that I wanted to live. They had gone through this and they were okay, and I wanted to be okay. I wanted to heal.

Joy. I've been fighting breast cancer for more than eight years. My journey started with a dream in August 1984. In the dream, I woke up in a recovery room in a hospital, and when I asked why I was there, a doctor said, "We removed your left breast because you have cancer." I told my friend and psychiatrist about my dream, and he urged me to get a mammogram and start doing self-exams.

I put off the mammogram because my husband was extremely ill with emphysema, and as his primary caregiver, I felt that I couldn't afford to worry about myself. I did start doing self-exams, and a couple of months later, I found a lump in my left breast. It was an elongated shape, and it seemed to me that a dangerous lump should be hard and round like a pea. The lump was also painful when I touched it, but I had fibrocystic disease, so I thought that must be what it was. I convinced myself that I was overreacting because of the dream. I kept delaying having the lump checked by my doctor.

Several months later my husband was well enough to return to work. I went to see my doctor on that very same day. He checked the lump, then sent me directly from his office to the hospital to have a mammogram. At that point, I knew it was cancer. That was just instinctive, not something I was told.

Two days later, the results were in, but because my doctor wanted my husband to be present when he told me the results of my mammogram, my appointment was delayed from three o'clock until four-thirty or five when my husband could get to the doctor's office. I stayed at work and waited. I resented having to wait. I knew what I was going to be told, and I wasn't worried—it was only cancer, it wasn't my life. That's what I thought the first three or four times I was diagnosed with cancer, and I honestly believed it at that time. This is only cancer, and I don't have time to mess with it. All I wanted was to go to my doctor's office and have him tell me what it was and get on with it. He had been caring for our family for fifteen years and was a friend. I was in total denial.

When I finally walked into my doctor's office late that afternoon, he was sitting there with my husband, and I could tell they'd already talked about my report. They looked at me with tears in their eyes. My primary reaction was, "Here are these two men and they already know; they have information about me which is very private. This is me. This is my thing." I felt so violated. I am a woman who wants to do things for herself. I wanted to say, "You had no right to discuss this without me. You had no right." If I was ever tempted to hit two people, it was right at that moment. My privacy had been invaded. I'm from a very large family—fifteen brothers and sisters—and, until I left home, the only space I ever had that was mine alone was one drawer in a bureau that nobody was allowed to touch. When I walked into my doctor's office and saw him and my husband looking at me that way, I felt as if they had opened my bureau drawer and dumped it out.

I didn't speak to my husband. I went directly back to work and continued to finish the calls I had planned for that day. I didn't intend to go home until I was ready. I worked until late that night, not knowing how to tell anyone or even if I wanted to tell anyone. After a week researching all the choices I had, I chose the biopsy with frozen sections. If cancer was confirmed, then the breast would be removed (a mastectomy) while I was still under the anesthetic.

I had a modified radical mastectomy. Out of twenty-one nodes, seven were positive and eleven were questionable. I went through nine or ten months of chemotherapy, then seven weeks of radiation. That was in 1985. Two years later I had severe, sharp pain in my left kidney. I was worried. I went through all the ultrasounds and every other test, and they couldn't locate it. Finally, with a bone scan, they discovered cancer in the second lumbar vertebra. A biopsy and a CT scan showed that it was a metastasis of my breast cancer. This was followed by seven weeks of radiation during which they also noted on the CT that there was a mass in the lower left lung. Additional testing confirmed metastatic activity in the lungs. At this point I thought, "Oh God, what next?" I kept remembering what the doctor had told me—"As long as the cancer is not in your soft tissues, as long as it doesn't get into your brain or your liver, you're okay. We'll keep you clear as long as we can." Before I was even done with that round of radiation, we discovered the lump in my right breast. And by this time I thought, "Where in the hell is this going to pop up next?" During this period of treatment and recovery from the lumpectomy (1988), my husband died. By 1990 it looked like this cancer period was behind me. Then in mid-1990, the fun began again. This time all of the lung activity, plus the right breast, became my new challenge!

The first time I was diagnosed with breast cancer, I felt that it was my body and my private affair. The second time and the third, I took my youngest son and my oldest daughter with me to hear the reports. They both listened for me and took notes. That worked well because I was now ready to share. The first diagnosis was horrible. After the second and third diagnoses I was able to cope so much better, even though I was getting bad news again. In retrospect, I believe that was due to my decision to allow those who loved me to share this experience with me.

⋙⋘

Daria. I found a lump in my breast in December 1991. It was very small, but it felt different, so I went for a mammogram. The mammogram showed no change from the one I'd had at age thirty-five, five years earlier, and they advised me to wait and have another mammogram in one year. In retrospect, I should have just had the lump removed—which is what I'd recommend to anyone now—but I was extremely busy with my work, and I didn't want to deal with the issue of, What if it's cancer? That summer, the lump changed acutely, suddenly becoming much larger and very painful. And I thought, "Hmmm, maybe it's a cyst or maybe it's not." A repeat mammogram in September showed microcalcifications that hadn't been there the year before. I knew in my heart that it would be cancer and scheduled myself for a visit to the surgeon, a wonderful woman who I greatly respect and who always shows such compassion to her patients. I was very frightened but didn't want to make a big deal out of it yet. My husband wanted to come with me for the initial visit, but I told him, "No, I need to treat this as a routine matter until such time as I know it's not routine." The biopsy was scheduled for the following week, and when the physician said, "It's malignant," my first thought was, "I'm dead." As an emergency room physician, I deal with people dying every day. My mother had died from breast cancer, and my grandmother had breast cancer. My mother lived only months after treatment. I immediately moved through all the possibilities and concluded, "That's it . . . I'm dead. Here it is September twenty-fourth, and this will be my last Christmas." I truly felt that way, even though I didn't yet have any lymph node stats or anything like that. I just thought, "Well, Daria, dead by Christmas."

⇌

Donna. In July 1990, I found a lump in my breast. A well-meaning physician told me it was a rib. When I asked why I didn't have a rib in the same place on the other side, he said not to worry. Six weeks later I sought a second opinion and was told I needed a biopsy. I asked my husband not to go with me. I said, "This is going to be a benign tumor. It's no big deal. I just need to go and get the information on it."

Following the biopsy, my physician walked into the room and said, "How are you?" I replied that I'd be just fine as soon as he gave me the good news. He said, "You have breast cancer." Then an oncologist came in and I turned to him and said, "I'm too young. I'm just thirty-six." I must have repeated that a dozen times—I'm too young.

In September I had a lumpectomy to remove the tumor, which was a two- to three-centimeter infiltrating ductal cancer. The nodes were negative, all the other scans were negative, and we were extremely pleased. I felt pretty positive about how things would go. Still I insisted that aggressive chemotherapy be done because of my age. So I had four cycles. A few weeks after I finished chemotherapy, I took off for Hawaii, and I felt great. My husband and I started traveling a lot. I lived every minute of the next two and a half years. I didn't let one go by me.

In January 1993 I started a high-impact aerobics class and began to have an increasing amount of back pain. I'd had back pain for twenty years, but this felt different. I continued the class, ignoring the pain. In March I started having rib pain. I thought, "This is not right." Lower back pain is one thing, but pinching pain in your rib is something else. I went to a radiation oncologist, and he told me, "Donna, you don't have bone disease. You look too good. You feel too good. The pain isn't bad. Don't worry. You don't have bone disease." Still, he agreed to a bone scan. Bless him for listening to me.

Once breast cancer has been found, more tests are done to determine if it has spread to other parts of the body, so that appropriate treatment can be planned. This process is called *staging*. The following stages are used for breast cancer.

Breast cancer in situ (also called carcinoma in situ) is very early cancer. There are two types of breast cancer in situ: ductal carcinoma (also called intraductal carcinoma) and lobular carcinoma (also called breast cancer in situ, carcinoma in situ, or Stage 0 breast cancer). Women diagnosed with lobular carcinoma in situ have a 25 percent chance of developing breast cancer in either breast within the next twenty-five years.

Stage I breast cancer is no larger than two centimeters (about one inch) and has not spread outside the breast.

Stage II breast cancer is no larger than two centimeters but has spread to the lymph nodes under the arm (the axillary lymph nodes); or the cancer is between two and five centimeters (from one to two inches) and may or may not have spread to the lymph nodes under the arm, or the cancer is larger than five centimeters (larger than two inches) but has not spread to the lymph nodes under the arm.

Stage IIIA breast cancer is smaller than five centimeters and has spread to the lymph nodes under the arm, and the lymph nodes are attached to each other or to other structures, or the cancer is larger than five centimeters and has spread to the lymph nodes under the arm.

Stage IIIB breast cancer has spread to tissues near the breast (skin or chest wall, including the ribs and muscles of the chest) or the cancer has spread to the lymph nodes inside the chest wall along the breastbone.

(continues)

(continued)

Stage IV breast cancer has spread to other organs of the body, most often the bones, lungs, liver, or brain, or the tumor has spread locally to the skin and lymph nodes inside the neck, near the collarbone.

Inflammatory breast cancer is a special class of rare breast cancer. With inflammatory breast cancer, the breast looks as if it is inflamed because of its red appearance and warmth. The skin may show signs of ridges and wheals or it may have a pitted appearance. Inflammatory breast cancer tends to spread quickly.

Treatment—Patients—Breast Cancer. Physician Data Query, Office of Cancer Communications, National Cancer Institute. April 1997 (last modified October 1996).

During the bone scan, I could tell something was wrong when I looked at the screen and saw the big bright spots. I knew. I told my husband, "Call my oncologist and tell him Donna is concerned. He'll understand. Get him over here." I couldn't believe that no radiologist, no physician at all, was present to interpret the bone scan. My oncologist arrived within twenty minutes. The diagnosis was metastatic breast cancer, bone disease. Three years ago, my primary diagnosis was very scary. This is different. This is anger more than fear.

2

Taking an Active Role

"I'm a person who has always controlled my own life, sometimes by choice, sometimes by necessity. I always need to feel that I'm in control of what is happening to me."

—*Joy Edwards*

First Steps to Regaining Control

At first, we couldn't think, couldn't absorb the information we were given. Our familiar internal resources abandoned us. For some of us, this feeling lasted a few hours; for others, it lasted days. In fact, that feeling—or at least the remembrance of that first feeling—is still with us and is often very disconcerting. Luckily, our backgrounds and training served us well. We began to regain control by reaching for the skills that have always been useful to us in our careers: time management, decisiveness, risk assessment, planning and problem solving, resource utilization, taking command and exercising authority, and delegation. We also began to reassert those personal attributes that

25

The diagnosis of breast cancer is an overwhelming blow for the majority of women. Compounding this is the necessity of making treatment decisions. Treatment is complex with a variety of options and outcomes. The two major treatment options, mastectomy and lumpectomy followed by adjuvant chemotherapy (given when all visible and known cancer has been removed by surgery or radiation), offer equivalent survival rates.

The usual methods of decision making used in business and other areas may not work for a woman diagnosed with a life-threatening illness.

Researchers selected forty-eight early-stage breast cancer patients to study the decision-making procedures used by breast cancer patients. They determined five empirical indicators that influence decision-making behavior: perceived salience of alternatives, conflict, information seeking, risk awareness, and deliberation.

Perceived salience refers to the extent to which the patient was aware of and attracted to a particular treatment option based upon information presented by the physician. The patient reframes the options in her own language and may add her own alternatives.

A choice is made based upon the understanding of the options. Subjects who responded to the salience of one option over another did not report conflict in their decision making or the need for further information or deliberation.

Decision conflict was reported when one of three conditions was present: when the patient had a treatment preference but was discouraged from considering it as viable; when the patient was unable to discriminate between treatment options; and when one treatment option was strongly recommended but it was not the patient's

(continues)

(continued)

preferred treatment. Subjects also reported conflict when they were pulled between their preferred treatment and the preference of their medical team and/or family.

Many patients defer quickly to their physicians' preference to end the conflict distress.

Information seeking occurred when patients were unable to discriminate among treatment alternatives and so began to seek outside information. Supportive information reduced conflict, nonsupportive information increased conflict.

Risk awareness patients were identified as either risk seeking or risk averse, depending on the amount of risk they were willing to take regarding treatment options. Deliberation occurred when patients considered more than one treatment option. The time needed for deliberation was related to the degree of conflict felt and the amount of information needed to relieve the conflict.

Pierce, P. "Deciding on Breast Cancer Treatment: A Description of Decision Behavior." *Nursing Research*. Jan/Feb. 42(1) (1993):22–28.

had always been there: energy, determination, composure, competence, and objectivity.

First we had to decide to "get going," to figure out what we were going to do about this diagnosis. That was the first, and biggest, step because it was difficult to decide to do something when we felt and believed we were on death's door—when we believed nothing we could do would make a difference. This feeling was an almost immobilizing symptom of our despair. Finally, the need to make a decision kicked in. We think it was habit. We're

thankful for it and gratified that our experience and training worked their way back to the surface of our thinking.

Our energy returned with the reassertion of our decision-making abilities, as did the determination to get
some organization into this mix and confusion of feelings
and facts. We, each in our own way, began to collect information from a variety of sources. We learned from
others and tried to fit what we learned into a framework
for approaching and resolving the problem. For some aspects of the dilemma, it was as simple as moving one set
of skills over to another arena of conflict, and to reducing
the conflict to distinct, manageable tasks.

Steps to regaining control:
- get the facts
- identify choices
- investigate consequences of choices
- consult experts
- network with peers (in this case, other women
  with breast cancer)
- establish an investigatory and support team
- evaluate treatment options against a set of personal
  and professional criteria such as personal tolerance
  levels, work responsibilities, professional persona,
  logistics and scheduling, importance of appearance

Strategies and Tactics for Regaining Control

We had to acknowledge our circumstances and go from
there. We each came up with ways to "put ourselves back
in the driver's seat." Cathy recounts, "At the time of my

recurrence, I found it disturbing to realize that all of the knowledge I had acquired about the lumpectomy and radiation I'd undergone three years earlier didn't apply to the mastectomy and reconstructive surgeries that now confronted me. This was a whole new ball of wax. Back to square one. I decided I'd better get going. For the second time, I hit the books and made telephone calls to the people I knew who could bring me up to snuff so I could feel equipped to make the decisions that I was facing." Sally says, "When I first got the diagnosis, I was shocked, but when the shock wore off, I said to myself, Okay, what are you going to do about this? I set out to gather all of the information I could find, sharing it openly with everyone and anyone in order to get their advice and help. I threw myself into this process. I needed to be in control of this disease." And Betsy relates, "Once I recovered from my initial shock, I took the skills I'd used in my practice of law and just moved them over to this new problem, assuming it could be attacked in a similar way."

Regaining a sense of control meant that we had to identify—even intuitively—those areas of the process over which we could exercise some choice.

Ways to exercise choice and regain control:

- choose your health-care team
- gather information and use available resources
- manage relationships with others
- focus on your personal needs first
- develop tactics to manage emotions
- don't hesitate to change physicians if you feel the need
- insist that your health-care team function as your consultants
- choose your physician(s) for follow-up care

Choosing a Health-Care Team

We began to reclaim control by immediately tackling the selection of our health-care team. We each asked, "What kind of physician do I want?" and set out to find one or more that made us feel comfortable and confident. We were fortunate to be able to choose our physician(s), rather than having the decision dictated by financial or insurance considerations.

Some of us chose not to be treated by the physician who had diagnosed us or who had done our biopsy. We gathered names from friends, women's groups, and cancer resource centers, then conducted interviews with physicians until we assembled a team willing to accommodate our needs for control and participation. We refused to be constrained when family or friends told us, "But this is the best doctor in town" or "This one is highly recommended."

We each felt that we were in charge of our own treatment, and none of us was willing to relinquish that control to medical experts. Some of us sought second and third opinions and some had to "fire" their physicians. Carol S. rejected two surgeons who she felt were overbearing. She wanted someone who would meet her head-on and whom she could imagine seeing for checkups once every three to six months for the rest of her life. Given the incredibly different options she received from different physicians, she realized that picking a surgeon and an oncologist was more art than science. She found that her skill in evaluating or even terminating a doctor transferred from the workplace to her "place" as a patient. Daria admits, "I know I often came across as being aggressive as gangbusters, but that's what I had to do to get where I am in my career. And if that's what it takes to deal with breast cancer, I'll do it."

When we found the right physician, it was worth the effort. Carol S. says about the surgeon she selected, "She didn't take me to the big formal office with the couch and the desk. We went into her examining room. It was just the two of us. She said, 'Having breast cancer is a bitch . . . What do you want to talk about?' She was right there. She felt familiar. She felt like home."

We had specific requirements for our health-care team in addition to clinical skill and knowledge about breast cancer. Some of us insisted that our physician be female; Daria selected "a physician who can look you right in the eye and be straight with you." Betsy sought "someone who is very knowledgeable and able to translate the medical information into understandable terms." And Joy looked for a physician "who doesn't object to being called by his/her first name . . . they can't hide behind the shield of 'Doctor So and So' . . . they're just Joe or Mary and we're consulting with each other." We all searched for a team that understood and accepted that we wanted them to be our consultants, not our bosses. As Joy explained to her physician, "You have medical knowledge about breast cancer that I don't have and what I need from you is information and options so I can make my decision."

We also chose the physician(s) we wanted to see for follow-up care. One of us regularly sees her surgeon, another keeps in contact with her oncologist, and one regularly consults her surgeon, oncologist, and radiologist. And some of us insist on having an oncologist on our follow-up team because cancer therapy is evolving and we want the most up-to-date information.

Identifying and Utilizing Information Resources

It was important for us to acknowledge that, even though the decisions were ours to make, outside resources were available to help us make those decisions. We contacted local cancer resource centers and national breast cancer groups to obtain ratings for physicians, to gather the most recent information about breast cancer, and to speak with survivors. We made connections with women's networks, requested literature searches, or visited medical libraries to conduct our own research. A few of us assembled teams of families and friends to whom we delegated research tasks. [Interestingly, as we will address in a later chapter, this proved to be an excellent strategy for occupying the time of those close to us whose distress might have been too emotionally overwhelming for us otherwise.]

As soon as she was diagnosed, Carol S. found herself assisted by a tight-knit team of researchers that included her son, her significant other, and three close women friends. One became an expert on oncology, one on chemotherapy, and one on radiation and surgery. They were all experienced researchers in their own professions and wedged these new tasks in with their regular responsibilities. Carol S.'s son, who was studying in England, flew home before her surgery and spent long hours with Carol and her partner at the University of San Francisco Medical School library weighing the pros and cons of lumpectomies versus mastectomies. Carol S. had to make her decision just before solid evidence hit the press on the relative safety of lumpectomies versus mastectomies. Despite her research the decision to have a lumpectomy was hard because she felt emotionally that it was a less aggressive response. Donna and Daria were very fortunate in that they were already involved in health-care delivery and had "inside" contacts who could provide the latest information on ongoing studies.

Some of us investigated the genetic link in breast cancer as part of our research. Daria tracked down her mother's oncologist in another part of the country to find out exactly what kind of cancer her mother had and why she had died so quickly after chemotherapy. The information she obtained helped her to make a decision about her own chemotherapy and helped her understand the implications for her own daughters.

Cathy recalls that in her research she found out about a breast cancer research laboratory that provides tumor banking, the storage of breast cancer tumor cells for use in future research. To participate, she had to arrange with her surgeon to ship her tumor to the lab. Her physician had no difficulty in complying with Cathy's request. Cathy feels that she, as well as others, may benefit from future research as a result of this arrangement.

The information we acquired and the resources we identified were indispensable, as was the help we received from our families and friends. Nonetheless, it was then, and still is, our responsibility to make the final decisions regarding our treatment—and to make it clear that they could be made neither by our physicians, our friends, our significant others, nor our families. This attitude comes, of course, from our being accustomed to making our own decisions and accepting the responsibility for those decisions in both our personal and professional lives. As Betsy says, "I'm constantly making decisions in my work, often decisions that are based on factors over which I have no control. When you make a lot of decisions, it's unrealistic to think you're not going to make mistakes. When I make a decision that turns out to be wrong, I accept responsibil-

Investigators have identified three styles of decision making. Patients were classified by their dominant decision-making style: deferrer, delayer, and deliberator.

Deferrers tended to be older (with a mean age of fifty-six) and generally made a quick treatment decision based on the immediate appeal of the option, or the opinion of their physician. They experienced little conflict or uncertainty and therefore little deliberation. Many subjects, in fact, did not have the experience of making a choice due to the strong salience of one option. Deferrers reported strong satisfaction with their choices and did not anticipate future regret.

Delayers structured their decision making in a way that allowed them to consider one or more options. Vacillation differentiated delayers from deferrers. Delayers appeared to jump from one option to the next and repeatedly compared options until one option clearly dominated. Delayers tended to be younger than deferrers.

Deliberators felt a personal responsibility for making a quality decision and took charge in a deliberate and purposeful manner. These patients are unique in that they expressed the following characteristics: They used a strategy or plan, explicitly considered risk, expressed confidence in their decision-making ability, and held a lingering uncertainty about the outcome. They anticipated that they may, at some time in the future, regret their choices.

Patients in this group tended to lay out a plan that identified the attributes of each treatment option, then gathered specific technical information and validated the information with expert opinions. Once this process began, it unfolded into an extensive information search designed to answer all treatment questions until one alternative satisfied most of the conditions.

(continues)

(continued)

Deliberators did not choose a treatment option until they were confident that they had all the pertinent information and had found a treatment option that satisfied their major needs.

These patients tried to minimize risks associated with treatment by gathering information about the treatments and by selecting the best medical team and treatment center. It was important for these patients to feel in control of the events in their lives and to identify those events that they could not control.

Conflict was an integral part of the decision-making process for deliberators. Although they reported feeling a sense of control over their decisions, they were also aware of the possibility of a negative outcome. Deliberators, unlike delayers and deferrers, did not express satisfaction with their choices, rather they used words such as *confidence* to describe their choices.

Deliberators armed themselves with an abundance of information before making a treatment choice. Many went against popular or professional opinion to get the treatment they preferred.

Deliberators experienced lingering doubts about their long-term outcomes—none was absolutely certain there was a best choice.

Of the three styles, deliberators are the closest to normative models of decision making; however, they experienced the greatest psychological distress. They spent the greatest amount of time, energy, and resources on their decision-making process.

Pierce, P. "Deciding on Breast Cancer Treatment: A Description of Decision Behavior." *Nursing Research*. Jan/Feb. 42(1) (1993):22–28.

ity. But no matter what happens, I feel comfortable with my decision because I know I made the best one I could at the time. I feel the same way about the choices I've made related to my breast cancer. I make the best decision I can. I'm prepared to deal with the consequences."

Meeting Our Own Needs First

It was important for us to conquer, or at least manage, our feelings of vulnerability. We are experienced in being viewed as "exceptionally competent," so this new sense of vulnerability and need was disquieting. We wanted to maintain an appearance of composure and strength, not only for our own sake, but also for the sake of those around us. Carol W. recalls, "I always felt that I had to be the strong one, the decision maker, that I always had to be there for others to lean on. So it was very difficult for me to involve anyone else in this process . . . to be open about my vulnerability."

We have learned that it is critical for us to place the highest priority on meeting our own needs before striving to satisfy the needs of others. Our experience in living with breast cancer has shown us the importance of time alone, privacy, and psychological space for us to wrestle with the physical, emotional, and psychological repercussions of this life-threatening illness.

It wasn't easy, however, to put our own needs first. We had a difficult time and often felt guilty. But as Joy and Cathy discussed, "There is a big difference between being selfish and being self-focused." We have come to realize that sometimes it is okay—even vital—to keep others at a distance while meeting our own needs and trying to come to terms with our illness. We have found that it is essential to give ourselves permission to focus on what is important to us, no matter how strange that sometimes feels. Once we had ourselves "in order," we found we could reach out to others to help them cope with our diagnosis.

As Joy says, "I've always been a person who believed that I had to put other people's needs ahead of my own. At first, I felt guilty about being selfish, for example, if I kicked everyone out of the bedroom, closed the door, and did my crying under the covers by myself. I have since been able to say, 'Joy, it's okay.'" For Daria, "There were periods when I needed to be alone. I needed time by myself to think through what was happening to me and to work it out. I had to feel free to be as emotional as I needed to be without worrying about how someone else was reacting."

An important aspect of our regaining control was deciding how much or how little interaction we wanted with our families and friends, then setting the parameters for that involvement. We identified our most intimate friends or "inner circle" and then educated them about what we needed and wanted in terms of emotional and physical support. It generally worked best for us to just clearly tell them how involved we wanted them to be. As Daria says, "I had a scare with bone pain and I was terrified that the cancer had metastasized. I asked my husband to come to the hospital with me for the bone scan, but we agreed ahead of time that he would not touch me. I didn't want him to put his arm around me, hold my hand, or touch me in any way. His role was simply to get me out of the building as quickly as possible if the news was bad. Part of my anxiety was the fear that I'd fall apart in front of other people. I wanted to maintain control of my emotions until I got home or at least until I reached the privacy of my car. So I asked my husband to run interference for me by not letting anyone stop me in the hall to talk."

We found that having to comfort distraught well-wishers was often troublesome and developed tactics for handling the well-wishers, often by transferring their concern to concrete action that could actually help us. We asked them to take notes during office visits, intercept phone calls, help us research new studies, and provide us with transportation to therapy.

We discovered that the ability to protect our privacy by placing limits on friends and family is a learned behavior and it isn't easy. We tried to protect our space, time, and privacy. But so many wonderful friends and colleagues called so often, and we felt guilty if we didn't call them back. It is very difficult to say no, but we're getting better at it! Carol H. recalls, "Because this was my second bout with cancer, friends were very supportive of whatever I needed. I chose to be the one to reach out when I needed to and to be left alone at other times."

Carol S. bought an answering machine for her telephone and installed a separate line with an unlisted number for use by her family and closest friends. She no longer answers her old number but simply picks up the messages when she is ready to deal with them. For Sally and Joy, mailing form letters to their friends and colleagues, letting them know how they were doing, and asking them not to call, worked best. Sally added a request that they send cards and prayers instead of calling.

The desire to keep friends and acquaintances at a manageable distance becomes particularly complicated in the event of recurrence. Donna recalls, "Following my initial diagnosis of breast cancer, I made the decision to satisfy my needs first and to keep all of those lovely people away from me. Now, since the recurrence, I struggle with the question of how long I should keep people away. I may need them when and if I become incapacitated. I just trust that if I need them later, they'll forgive me for keeping them at a distance before."

Controlling Our Emotions

Another facet of reclaiming control involved finding ways to cope with the emotional roller coaster on which we sometimes found ourselves. We feared the loss of emotional control, especially in front of colleagues and subordinates. We wanted to manage our circumstances to ensure that we had privacy when we became emotional or when we heard bad news.

Breast cancer is an emotional experience, but most of our work environments are not amenable to emotional expression—we feel we have to hold back, wait for an appropriate time, a private time, to let it out. Many of us have spent years sublimating our emotions in order to function efficiently and be professional. But, for some of us, if we can't express our emotions, we tend to suppress them, and we even forget how to *feel* at all.

Managing emotions:
- find a "safe" place to cry
- try to control when and how you receive your test results
- try meditation, visualization, or complementary techniques

It is important to release emotions, to cry, but we have learned that there are places and circumstances where it is just not appropriate to display our feelings. All of us find it uncomfortable to cry "in public." And, of course, the workplace is usually the most inappropriate place for crying. There is only a small circle of people with whom we feel comfortable crying. For some of us, that circle included our support groups. When we received the news of our diagnosis, we sought a safe and private place to "let go."

Perhaps the most devastating event in having breast cancer is hearing the diagnosis for the first time. But there are other points during the course of breast cancer that are also very difficult—waiting for the results from biopsies, metastatic workups following mastectomies, follow-up bone scans, and other tests.

We often found it difficult to control our fear and anxiety during those times, so it helped to control how and when we received reports. For example, Daria asked her surgeon to give her the results of her lymph node biopsies over the phone so that she could process the information privately before seeing the surgeon. She received the results on Friday, two days after her mastectomy. In retrospect, she thinks she should have just told her surgeon to wait until Monday to tell her because she didn't see the point of hearing what could be bad news a few days earlier when there was nothing she could do about it. She could have had the weekend to focus on recovering from surgery.

Some of us found we could decrease our anxiety by getting our test results as quickly as possible. Donna found she became impatient with the medical staff when her test results were delayed, so she found a confidential telephone number for laboratory and X-ray results. She now calls for her results herself. This gives her time to deal with them so she can be ready when she talks with her physician.

Since Sally lives only a couple of blocks from the hospital, she walks to the hospital on the day the reports are supposed to be ready and gets her own copy. This gives her enough information to figure out what questions she wants to ask her physicians.

Controlling our fear of recurrence is a continuing challenge. Some of us have found that meditation or visualization helps to manage fear and anxiety. As Donna says, "Talk about maintaining control! Knowing that I can lower my level of anxiety in the midst of an extremely stressful situation makes me feel incredibly powerful."

We know that control has different meanings for each of us. For Carol H. "Control . . . is associated with making the people around me feel good. I am a great listener, and my concern for others helps divert my attention from myself. And that was one way I took back my control." And for Betsy, "Advocacy is extremely important to me because it provides me with the opportunity to do something that might make a difference in terms of breast cancer. My advocacy work has given me a great deal of satisfaction, and it has made me feel a little better about having breast cancer. I feel a little more in control."

3

Deciding About Treatment

"It was time to think fast. I decided to take the big gun approach—to hit it hard and heavy."
—**Daria Davidson**

Once we moved beyond the shock of diagnosis, we acted decisively. We researched the medical literature, interviewed physicians, solicited second opinions, and sought out survivors of breast cancer for firsthand accounts. Armed with this information, we then searched our own minds and hearts before making the difficult decision of choosing a therapy. For some of us, the type of therapy was dictated by the location, size, and estrogen receptor status of our tumors; lymph node involvement; and/or our history of cancer. We all had the choice of whether to pursue medical treatment.

The decision about the type of therapy took some of us a few days, others a few weeks, and some even longer. We didn't agonize over our decisions, but we did do our homework and gave it due attention. We felt strongly that we needed to be "allowed" to control the process to meet our own schedules and information needs. For example, it was about a month from Carol S.'s biopsy until her surgery; for Betsy it was about ten days; and Daria moved fast—because she is a physician, choosing a physician and evaluating treatment options proved easier for her.

Some of us were encouraged by our physicians to take our time in reaching our decisions. Carol W. found it reassuring that her physician wanted her to take her time. Others of us felt pushed or rushed but ultimately took the time we believed we needed, despite pressure from our physicians. We weighed a number of factors during our decision-making process, including the success rate for each treatment in terms of recurrence (disease-free interval) and survival; our ability to tolerate the side effects of treatments, such as chemotherapy and radiation; changes in physical appearance and their effect on body image; time away from work and our ability to function effectively during the treatment phase; and the flexibility of the treatment regimen, that is, our ability to control the scheduling of treatments to minimize disruption to our work and personal lives.

Choosing the kind of therapy involved both medical and emotional considerations. Some of us were afraid of the surgery itself; others thought it would "get it [the cancer] all and be done with it." We were particularly concerned about our ability to handle chemotherapy—we had all heard horror stories. And paramount in our deliberations was the need—deep and pervasive—to feel confident and convinced that the treatments we chose would cure us of the cancer.

Our decision-making processes included contacting other women who had survived breast cancer. Carol H. believes that talking to breast cancer survivors brought her to a stage of believing that she wanted to fight the disease and live. After listening to women who had gone through the necessary medical treatments and were okay, she decided that she was willing to do the same. Carol S.

maintained telephone contact with several breast cancer survivors and considers them "incredibly generous and caring. They called back twenty times if that's what it took to reach me."

Lumpectomy or Mastectomy

Following our initial diagnoses, eight of us had lumpectomies and two had mastectomies. We each evaluated the medical literature and made our own judgment about whether breast-conserving therapy was as effective in preventing recurrence as was mastectomy.

Issues surrounding lumpectomy and mastectomy:

- the best "protection" against recurrence
- a sense of normalcy—avoiding a visual reminder
- appearance: not wanting friends and colleagues to wonder
- to reconstruct or not to reconstruct: another option or just another decision?
- recovery time

In addition to medical considerations, a number of other factors influenced our choice of either mastectomy or lumpectomy. Emotional issues were important; we considered things such as the effect physical changes would have on our sense of ourselves and on our husbands, significant others, and even colleagues. We wondered how we would deal with the disfigurement resulting from a mastectomy, a visible daily reminder of cancer and our own vulnerability. Daria says, "I finally decided that the stress of having a mastectomy, with the constant

Although lumpectomy plus radiation has been determined to be equally efficacious as mastectomy in the treatment of early-stage breast cancer, the majority of women undergoing breast cancer treatment opt for mastectomy.

Among women given a choice between lumpectomy and mastectomy, younger women who were more concerned about body image were more likely to choose lumpectomy.

Lazovick, D., White, E., Thomas, D., et al. "Underutilization of Breast-Conserving Surgery and Radiation Therapy among Women with Stage I or II Breast Cancer." *Journal of the American Medical Association.* 266(24) (1991):3433–38.

reminder of cancer every time I looked in the mirror, would be less than the stress due to my worrying about whether a lumpectomy had gotten it all."

It was important for us to maintain a sense of normalcy, and to look and feel natural. Choosing a lumpectomy usually allows a quick return to work because it typically involves a shorter recovery time and less likelihood of decreased arm mobility. A few of us reasoned that by choosing lumpectomy, we could reserve the more drastic step of mastectomy as an option if the cancer recurred. In fact, this did happen to Cathy. She chose to have a lumpectomy at the time of her initial diagnosis of breast cancer, and when the cancer recurred three years later, she had a mastectomy with immediate reconstruction.

Two other factors that we weighed in our decision were our stage and type of cancer and the risk of recurrence based on our family history of the disease. Daria chose to have a mastectomy, in part because she had an aggressive tumor similar to the kind that had killed her mother.

> A prospective evaluation of 109 newly diagnosed breast cancer patients who had received either mastectomy or breast-conserving surgery found no significant difference in mood, quality of life, or psychosocial adjustment between the groups at one year after surgery, with the exception of problems with body image and clothing.
>
> Patients receiving lumpectomy reported greater initial distress at one month, possibly due to the more rigorous radiation therapy. At six months postsurgery this distress had declined significantly. By one year distress was at a minimal level equal to that of the mastectomy patients.
>
> Ganz, P., Coscarelli-Shag, A., Lee, J. J., et al. "Breast Conservation versus Mastectomy." *Cancer.* 69(7) (1992):1729–38.

Reconstruction

Two of us who had mastectomies had immediate breast reconstruction. Although Joy wanted to have immediate reconstruction and had a plastic surgeon present during her mastectomy, she was not a candidate for the additional surgery. A year after completing radiation and chemotherapy, when reconstruction was possible, she decided, "It wasn't worth the effort. I had lived with me like this for that long and I didn't want additional surgery."

Daria and Cathy viewed the ability to have immediate reconstruction as an important aspect of their emotional recovery from breast cancer. In particular, it gave them another focus during the surgery and treatment process. Both found their encounters with their plastic surgeons positive and encouraging. Daria remembers, "Deciding to have an immediate reconstruction was absolutely the best decision I made. My desire for this procedure was at least twofold: If I didn't have it done before chemotherapy, I would have had to wait until after chemo to have it done; also, my visual image of a mastectomy is that of mutilation. By immediately beginning reconstruction, my internal self-esteem needs would be better met. The plastic surgeon inserted a prosthesis made of a combination of silicon and saline (a saline bladder with a thin layer of silicone on the outside). I had a small breast mound immediately after surgery, which was inflated every week. It gave me something else to focus on. My visits to the plastic surgeon were positive experiences compared to the other things I was going through. My husband got quite involved, and the doctor always let him do the inflating of my breast, so we all had some good laughs at a time when they were very much needed. I felt better because other people didn't feel quite so sorry for me." Cathy

---

A study of women undergoing either immediate or delayed reconstruction found that patients electing immediate reconstruction admitted to more concerns about their feelings of femininity, sexuality, and body symmetry than those choosing delayed reconstruction.

The immediate reconstruction group also reported fewer depression symptoms, fewer feelings of being deformed after mastectomy, and less discomfort. The immediate reconstruction group described their new breast as a restoration or replacement for the lost breast.

Stevens, L., McGrath, M. H., Druss, R. G., et al. "The Psychological Impact of Immediate Breast Reconstruction for Women with Early Breast Cancer." *Plastic and Reconstructive Surgery.* 73(4) (1984):619–26.

says, "I had a lot of questions when I found myself facing breast cancer a second time, and this time mastectomy surgery was the recommended course to take. Three years earlier, I had been told that, should a mastectomy be required, it would be one year before a reconstructive surgeon could build me a new breast. I didn't even realize that in the three years since that time, things had changed in the medical arena, and that many women were now considered candidates for 'immediate' breast reconstruction. I was absolutely thrilled when my surgeon explained the new procedure to me, and I realized I wouldn't have to wait a year to reconstruct my breast. I had wondered how well I would cope with enduring one year with an external prosthesis and realize now how little I knew, and that I had a lot of homework to do in researching the treatment options that faced me. I was delighted that the three years had afforded the benefit of different surgical options. For me . . . there was never any question that I wanted to do everything possible to bring my body back to symmetry and as natural an appearance as science and medical technique could provide."

Cathy says that both times she faced breast cancer, the possibility of disfigurement was a serious concern to her, and this concern affected her choice of surgeries and other treatment options. She didn't consider her disease life threatening, mainly because she was diagnosed in its earliest stage. She believed she had the "luxury" of concerning herself with what others may view as secondary matters, such as disfigurement and changes in her body symmetry and body image. She learned, however, that reconstruction "immediately after surgery" really means that you wake up from surgery with a breast mound "under construction." Both Cathy and Daria felt that the reconstruction, including reconstruction of the nipple, was

There are several types of reconstruction procedures which utilize a woman's own tissue, including the myocutaneous flap and the free-gluteus flap reconstruction. The myocutaneous flap involves a flap of muscle, fat, and skin which is removed from the back or abdomen. The tissue is moved in a sort of mound, under the skin to the area of the mastectomy. It remains attached via a feeding artery and vein to the old site. That site is stitched closed. Because the blood flow is maintained it may feel more "natural" than an implant although there is a definite reduction in sensation. The flap surgery usually requires a hospital stay of four or five days, and a recovery period of up to six weeks.

The free-gluteus flap is a very difficult and complex surgery. For this type of reconstruction, the tissue, skin, and muscle are taken from the buttocks. The blood supply cannot be maintained because of the distance from the gluteus to the chest, so the veins and blood vessels are cut and reconnected with the veins and blood vessels in the chest. The operation is long, with a hospital stay of about seven days. Because the blood supply is cut off there is a possibility of part of the flap dying, which will necessitate further surgery.

Love, S. *Dr. Susan Love's Breast Book*. 2nd edition. Addison-Wesley Publishing Company, Inc. Reading, Mass. 1995, pp. 392–94.

an important aspect in their retaining their positive self-esteem and self-image.

Typically, breast reconstruction with an implant is a three-step process, involving three surgeries (the final surgery being nipple-areola reconstruction, which some women opt to omit). This type of breast reconstruction is sometimes the only option available to those who don't have enough extra skin and body fat necessary for "flap" surgery.

For reconstruction with an implant, an inflatable tissue-expander device replaces the removed breast during the initial surgery. Shortly after the mastectomy comes the first tissue expansion, during which the device is inflated and the new mound actually grows in size. The purpose of the tissue expansion process is to stretch the skin to accommodate a permanent breast implant.

Cathy chose to have immediate reconstruction with a silicone implant. The process involves inserting under the skin a tissue expander that is gradually inflated to the desired size. An implant then surgically replaces the expander. As Cathy explains, "The homework I had done on mastectomy/reconstructive surgeries had helped me to understand that I didn't need to find the greatest breast surgeon in the world—I knew that breast reconstruction was not a particularly complicated surgery; many reconstructive surgeons in town could certainly build me a nice-looking breast. . . . What I was looking for was a doctor I felt I could communicate with, and I found that. All in all, the expansion process went by quickly, and I selected a silicone gel–filled implant with a textured silicone shell on the exterior, as the gel had the most natural feel and weight to it, and the research seemed to indicate that the textured exterior decreased capsular contracture. My surgeries took place about a year prior to the implant controversy, with which I subsequently became quite involved." Cathy has testified on the pro-implant side of the issue for state legislators and was interviewed on ABC's *Nightline*. Others of us feel equally strongly about the negative aspects of the use of silicone implants for breast reconstruction after mastectomy.

Radiation and/or Chemotherapy

Our decisions to have radiation therapy, chemotherapy, or both were based on a number of factors but primarily on our desire to "do it all" and/or the ability to fit one or both into our busy and demanding work schedules.

On chemotherapy:

- choose a regimen that fits best into your professional schedule and lifestyle
- ask about clinical trials
- find out when and for how long side effects will occur
- be prepared for the worst
- you can decide how flexible your treatment schedule will be
- investigate self-care techniques such as exercise, meditation, and diet alterations to minimize intensity of side effects
- consider appearance enhancements (makeup, wig, scarves, etc.)

While we wanted to do everything we could in terms of treatment, we were not willing to undergo therapies that were not sensible or logical for our particular diagnoses.

When radiation was presented as the option of choice, we all agreed to have radiation, even though it involved an arduous schedule of treatments nearly every day for six weeks. When the physician presented a choice of radiation or chemotherapy, the decision was more difficult. Some of us chose to do both out of a desire to "do it all

Advances in detection and treatment options for cancer patients have improved the five-year survival rates for many cancers, including breast cancer. The focus of cancer treatments has recently expanded to include the issue of quality of life for cancer patients. Patients must weigh the costs, both in survival outcome and emotional distress, with the benefits of treatment. The FDA now includes quality of life after treatment as one of the main criteria by which new cancer treatments are judged for approval.

Each aspect of cancer treatment—diagnosis, surgery, radiation, and chemotherapy—has an impact on all areas of a patient's life. Each brings concerns and fears about the impact of the treatment on quality of life.

Surgery for breast cancer may bring about acute stress. Many patients fear they will never awaken from the anesthesia. Breast cancer patients face the loss of a very personal part of their bodies, one that symbolizes both their femininity and maternity. These factors impact the patient both physically and emotionally.

Radiation side effects may include fatigue, decrease in appetite, burns, and in some patients anorexia and loss of libido. Radiation also requires a major time commitment for many breast cancer patients, involving daily visits to the hospital for extended periods of time.

Chemotherapy is often the most feared aspect of cancer treatment. The side effects are well known, and they are viewed by many cancer patients as being the most vivid reminder of their illness. Side effects may include nausea, weight gain or loss, fatigue, diarrhea, mouth sores, sleep disturbances, and loss of hair.

While the effects of these treatments on quality of life can be generalized to some extent, each individual has special needs and concerns that need to be considered when making treatment decisions.

Cella, D. "Quality of Life during and after Cancer Treatment." *Comprehensive Therapy.* 14(5) (1988):69–75.

and make sure it wouldn't come back." We believe our individual decisions were a result of both the recommendations of our physicians and our own level of comfort with uncertainty and risk. Some of us really wanted "closure—this is the problem, this is how to solve it, now we can put it aside." Others of us wanted "a reserve" and we selected a "one step at a time" approach. In retrospect, we know we were afraid of the treatments, but our fears really did not seem to be a factor in our decision. For each of us, the fear of recurrence was the major factor.

Our primary concern about chemotherapy was whether we would feel well enough to function at work during the months of treatment. Many of us were, and are, accustomed to feeling tired and stressed, a function of our professional lives, so these side effects were not particularly worrisome to us. But we knew nausea would be a significant problem. It is one thing to say, "I didn't miss a day of work," but nausea and vomiting on the job are not the glamorous, "do-it-all" image we had in mind for ourselves. We had also heard about anticipatory nausea—getting sick just thinking of how sick chemotherapy can make you—so we knew it could be really bad.

Our concerns about possible side effects influenced our choices of chemotherapeutic regimen. More potent chemotherapeutic agents, higher doses, and more intense regimens (three months versus six months) are associated with more severe side effects. The route of administration—intravenous or oral—affects the flexibility of scheduling the regimen into the workday. We had to weigh our desire to treat the cancer as aggressively as possible against the regimen's impact on our professional responsibilities and our personal lifestyles. For Daria, "Aside from the fear of death, chemotherapy was my big issue. My biggest fear from the beginning was whether I'd be able to handle the chemotherapy. I knew that people get really sick on chemotherapy, and I didn't want to be that sick, especially if it wasn't going to make much difference in terms of my survival. I decided that if the lymph nodes came back negative, then chemotherapy was probably worth it to me. If it turned out there was cancer in most of the nodes taken, then I didn't want to fight a battle with those kind of odds."

We chose our own chemotherapy regimens and lived through those choices. Our physicians gave us options based on our personal and professional lifestyles. And it was important for us to know, ahead of time, about the most adverse side effects of the regimen so we could evaluate how it would affect our ability to carry out our professional and social responsibilities—"Prepare me for the worst; I can work backward from there!" Considerations included time commitment versus intensity (three-month intense versus six-month extended, for example); how treatments would be administered and the time commitment required for individual treatments; time to onset of vomiting and/or nausea—"Should I schedule for the first thing in the morning and miss one day of work, or the last thing in the evening and try to struggle through the next day at work?"—and self-care options to help get us through treatment, such as diet alterations, homeopathic remedies, acupuncture, and exercise. Some of us had health-care professionals who worked with us to establish flexible treatment schedules to fit in with our personal and professional schedules. Others were not so fortunate. None of us had to make choices that newly diagnosed women today must make in light of recent reports that show significant success with chemotherapy and/or radiation treatment prior to surgery.

Because Daria had only a tiny spot in one of her nodes, she was given a choice of having the standard six months

Recent studies in lung cancer patients have demonstrated a significant increase in survival time for patients given preoperative chemotherapy. Researchers now suggest that induction chemotherapy for locally advanced solid tumors, such as breast cancers, may, theoretically, offer several advantages. Chemotherapy is tolerated with more ease, allowing for more aggressive therapy; shrinkage of the tumor may increase the likelihood of resection and complete elimination within the radiation field; treatment is begun immediately for all cancer sites, both those that are visible on CAT scans and microsites that are too small to be detected with currently available means; and, finally, chemotherapy is more active against untreated, locally advanced cancers than against metastatic disease.

Green, M. R. "Multinodal Therapy for Solid Tumors." *New England Journal of Medicine.* 330(3) (1994):206–7.

of CAF (Cytoxan, Adriamycin, 5-FU) or participating in one of the clinical trials for women with one to three positive nodes. The clinical trial regimen involved "big gun" heavy-duty intravenous doses that cause severe nausea and vomiting, but only for three months instead of the usual six. She considered the three-month regimen because it would allow her to return to her work in patient care in a shorter amount of time. She talked with some physician friends and then decided it would be better to try the clinical trial. "Once I decided to have chemotherapy, my fear of it stopped being an issue. I decided to take the big gun approach—hit it hard and heavy, and be really sick but for a shorter amount of time." Her main focus was on getting rid of the disease, within preestablished "tolerance" parameters, and she pushed these parameters to the limit.

Like Daria, Joy also chose to participate in a clinical trial, in part because she also liked the idea of being closely followed by physicians for several years. Others of us decided against enrolling in clinical trials because we viewed the inflexibility of the protocol as a loss of control over our treatment. We were not willing to commit ourselves to a single course of action, preferring to maintain the ability to direct our own care, especially if new therapies became available. In spite of trends that have made clinical trials more available, the American Cancer Society estimates that only 4 percent of newly diagnosed cancer patients enroll in clinical trials.

We must be honest. Chemotherapy was a truly unpleasant experience. Some of us had it worse than others. A few of us lost all our hair, and we generally looked "green," probably because we felt sick. Some of us went through violent bouts of vomiting, although those who took antinausea medication found some relief. We had difficulty concentrating at work and sometimes experienced a vague "fuzziness."

Tamoxifen

Four of us chose to take tamoxifen. Sally took tamoxifen on a three-month trial basis. Because her estrogen receptor status was negative, her physician suggested it, hoping to avoid the chemotherapy that Sally was so against. It didn't work at all. She says, "My cancer grew beautifully on tamoxifen." Donna has taken tamoxifen for metastatic disease and relates that "it stabilized my disease and I've had no side effects."

Betsy's doctor advised her to take tamoxifen after she completed her chemotherapy. However, she says, "I de-

Tamoxifen has been hailed as the miracle cure for breast cancer recurrence. While researchers argue about how it works—by binding with the estrogen receptors on the cell, by neutralizing an enzyme that is part of the cancer causing mechanism, or by starving the cells of the estrogen they need to grow—physicians are prescribing it for more and more women. Many young women are currently being given the "entire scope of treatment" including chemotherapy, radiation, and tamoxifen. Tamoxifen, while less toxic than other chemotherapy drugs, does have side effects, which may include nausea, rash, premature menopause and, in some cases, an increased risk for endometrial cancer.

LaTour, K. *The Breast Cancer Companion.* William Morrow and Company, Inc. New York, 1993, pp. 173–74.

cided not to take it at that time because I was premenopausal and because I wanted to take one treatment at a time. I also wanted to give my body a chance to establish the new normalcy."

Joy was on tamoxifen therapy from September 1985 through October 1990. She experienced headaches on the first dosage level. The headaches became less pronounced when the dosage was reduced. When renewed activity of her lung cancer occurred in October 1990, tamoxifen therapy was discontinued.

Carol W. did not choose to take tamoxifen, though her doctor prescribed it. Her doctor told her that it was the only thing that seemed to control recurrence. It was not the cure, but it was the best preventive medicine available at the time. Not having had to take medications for any reason, she resisted the notion of being subjected to this drug for an undetermined length of time. She also resisted

Clinical trials have begun to determine whether tamoxifen can prevent the development of breast cancer. The rationale for this study is based upon evidence that tamoxifen interferes with the initiation and development of breast cancer, clinical evidence of decreased development of breast cancer in the normal breasts of women participating in tamoxifen clinical trials for breast cancer, and the low toxicity of tamoxifen as compared with other chemotherapeutic agents. Tamoxifen has also been found to prevent the loss of bone density in postmenopausal women and to lower serum cholesterol levels.

If tamoxifen is to be used as a chemopreventative for breast cancer development, the safety of the drug in a cancer-free population must be of paramount importance. Although the side effects of tamoxifen are few, they do exist. Included are the possibility of increased endometrial cancer, other second generation cancers, and thromboembolytic events. Researchers will need to investigate the potential risk-to-benefits ratio and weigh the cost of lives saved versus the potential for serious side effects.

Chelbowski, R. T., Butler, J., Nelson, A., et al. "Breast Cancer Chemoprevention." *Cancer.* 72 (1993):1032–37.

this additional intrusion in her life and put off filling the prescription for six weeks. She relented just before beginning her radiation treatments. As she says, "I still haven't fully accepted this type of control over my life and occasionally I 'forget' to take a pill. The only side effect I have experienced is a little weight gain."

Carol S. relates her experience with deciding whether to take tamoxifen: "I didn't begin taking tamoxifen immediately after I finished six months of chemotherapy and seven weeks of radiation. Several members of my support group had terrible reactions to tamoxifen, and it made sense to me to wait a couple of months and get my body and mind somewhat cleared of the impact from the chemo and radiation. That way I could have a baseline for whatever my reaction to tamoxifen would be. And then there is my general resistance to any drugs, especially those that doctors automatically put you on, like their bias for prescribing hormone therapy for women of a certain age. My doctor just assumed I would go right on tamoxifen but agreed with my argument to take a break. He did warn me that the studies on the benefits of the drug are based upon women beginning tamoxifen immediately after chemo (in a case like mine) and that he did not know what difference a break in treatment would make. Planetree, a nonprofit cancer resource library in

Tamoxifen is a drug that blocks the effects of estrogen in the breast. Because of this action, it has been studied extensively in the treatment of breast cancer. A recent study of about 3,000 women showed that the women diagnosed with primary operable breast cancer who had estrogen-positive tumors and no axillary node involvement who received five years of tamoxifen therapy benefited significantly. The women who received tamoxifen had longer disease-free survival and fewer developed cancer in the other breast than did those who did not receive the drug. Women under 49 as well as those over 50 benefited equally from tamoxifen therapy. Studies with tamoxifen are ongoing in women with breast cancer and women who are disease free.

Fisher, B., Dignam, J., Bryant, J., et al. Five versus more than five years of tamoxifen therapy for breast cancer patients with negative lymph nodes and estrogen receptor–positive tumors. *Journal of the National Cancer Institute.* 88(21) (1996): 1529–42.

A recent case-control study supports the hypothesis that tamoxifen taken after breast cancer increases the risk for endometrial cancer. Of the ninety-eight patients diagnosed with endometrial cancer at least three months after the diagnosis of breast cancer, 24 percent were taking tamoxifen. The study also found that the risk for developing endometrial cancer increased with the amount of time the patients used the drug. For the women taking tamoxifen for more than two years, the risk of developing endometrial cancer was two times greater than for the women who had never taken the drug.

van Leeuwen, F. E., Bendraadt, J., Coebergh, J. W. W., et al. "Risk of Endometrial Cancer after Tamoxifen Treatment of Breast Cancer." *The Lancet.* 343 (8895) (1994):448–52.

San Francisco, did a search of the literature for me, and I took the abstracts of articles on the pros and cons of tamoxifen to my surgeon, radiologists, and oncologist and asked them to review the latest findings with me. Just as I expected, their opinions were different, and in the end it is just like the beginning, trying to decide what kind of treatment to follow. The decision is mine."

When Breast Cancer Recurs

In choosing therapy, we analyzed many different factors. Ultimately, we put aside our fears of surgery, radiation, and chemotherapy, and our concerns about the impact of particular treatments on our ability to continue working, and selected the treatment we believed offered us the best chance for survival.

Anxieties during treatment:

- survival will be your main concern and will influence your choice of treatments
- no one can guarantee that your cancer will not recur or metastasize
- fears about recurrence can be tempered by keeping current on research developments
- recurrence does not mean you have to relinquish control or your right to choose your treatment

Survival was and is our overriding concern. We wanted our physicians to do whatever it took to cure us, and then send us home and tell us we'd never have to worry about this disease again. That was really all we cared about. But physicians cannot give those assurances, and, on our darker days, treatment seemed to be just another awful step in an inevitable process. The question of "when will this cancer come back" was always with us.

Four of us did have recurrences or experienced metastasis. Donna's cancer metastasized to her bones, Sally's had metastasized to the lymph nodes in her abdomen, and Joy's cancer metastasized to her other breast, as well as her lungs and bones. Cathy's cancer recurred in the same breast. Sally and Donna, statistically, had low risk for recurrence or metastasis, but both of their cancers metastasized—Sally's to the lymph nodes of the abdomen, and Donna's to her spine. Sally believes her cancer had already metastasized before her primary diagnosis. Two years after the removal of her left breast, Joy's cancer metastasized to her lumbar vertebrae and then her lungs. Two years later, a tumor developed in her right breast and she chose to have a second mastectomy.

Dealing with the fear of recurrence or metastasis:

- check out each possible symptom or sign
- be prepared for high stress when symptoms occur
- use past experience to help determine how you will cope with new information

We know we will always have a nagging fear of recurrence and metastasis. A pain here, a pinch there, or a bump somewhere else never goes unnoticed. Not surprisingly, we find that, even now, we let our pains continue for a while before checking them out with a physician. Joy always lives with a sign or symptom for one week; if it is still present at the end of that time, she calls her physician and checks it out. In a sense, our waiting is a type of denial—after all, the statistics are pretty good for women with Stage I or II breast cancer. And we think of ourselves—it's a holdover—as being risk taking rather than risk averse.

But we ultimately return to our physicians to check out any warning sign. We're learning. Daria describes her return visit as "the second worst moment after the initial diagnosis and node evaluation." She developed back pain and had a CT scan—and could tell immediately from the look on the radiation technologist's face that everything was okay. However, when Donna had her bone scan, she could tell from the technologist's behavior that the results were not good.

Even if cancer has metastasized, there are options for treatment. Those of us who have not had a recurrence or metastasis can only guess about how we would react or feel if our cancer returned: "I would continue fighting because the last two experiences have taught me that I can really handle anything"; "I probably will consider myself dead—and may not opt for further treatment"; "I'm sort of resigned; it makes me tired to think about it—and I'm not sure if I would even tell my husband and family."

Donna and Sally are currently dealing with metastasis after a node-free early diagnosis. The spectrum of their emotions and actions ranged from intense fear and anger followed by deep sadness to a reinvestigation of options, this time moving further into complementary therapies and soul-soothing strategies. They admitted to being forced to "cut back"—to reduce activities (not necessarily their work schedules) so they now have time for meditation, visualization, relaxation techniques, and stress reduction exercises.

On primary diagnosis, Donna and her husband refused to let cancer become the big thing in their lives—the cancer was just a small part of her, it did not define her. But once the cancer metastasized, she "allowed" it, by necessity, to assume a bigger role in her mental, physical, and spiritual life. She has been forced to pay attention to it and has actually used it to find out more about herself and about life. This is admittedly a hard way to learn what many people will never learn, but for Donna there is solace in this approach. She also has found that there are very special pleasures in life—travel, fine wine, an evening talking with her husband, a long phone call with her sister, buying a new car. "I love my husband so much. I love a good bottle of Chardonnay, too. . . . Everything I feel these days seems more intense than what I was capable of before. I've grown spiritually, and this experience is just sort of filling me up, but I wonder when I'm just going to stop. One wouldn't think that you could carry on with this level of emotional vigor forever."

Donna continues, however, actively to pursue traditional treatment. Her physician has given her drugs to suppress her hormone function, and she has had her ovaries removed. She is now undergoing treatment with one of the aggressive chemotherapy protocols. She has set a date for a stem-cell transplant that will occur if her current therapy goes well. As a result, she has resigned her current position but will return to her company in a new role.

Sally is further along in her treatment for metastatic disease and has undergone a stem-cell transplant. Her focus is not only on trying therapies (traditional or complementary) that have shown some substantive results in the research, but also on filling her life with the things she most enjoys doing. Like Donna, Sally has specific activities she greatly enjoys such as skiing and scuba diving. She measures life's events and schedules her treatments according to her scuba and skiing trips. ("I was skiing when . . ."; "I delayed my chemo until after my scuba diving trip . . .")

Both Donna and Sally read extensively about breast cancer, and both are involved in breast cancer activities: Sally is involved with support groups and Donna with the National Breast Cancer Coalition. Sally has changed the focus of her academic research because of her experience with breast cancer. She now focuses on the psychosocial issues related to breast cancer.

Cathy also deals with her recurrence on a daily basis because *The Home Show* (the television program that she helps produce) presents the latest updates on breast cancer as they occur. Joy has dealt with breast cancer recurrence and metastasis for the longest period of time (since 1987), and we all learn from her.

For some of us, recurrence is probably related to what we consider misdiagnoses when our primary tumors were discovered. Misdiagnoses are not uncommon, and it is important to be alert to that fact when analyzing disease status and treatment options.

Sally, Donna, Joy, and Cathy had, and continue to have, numerous and varied options for treating their disease. As each did with her initial therapy for breast cancer, each again went through a process when the cancer recurred of gathering information, analyzing data, and consulting with numerous physicians before selecting a therapeutic approach.

Complementary Therapeutic Choices

Each of us chose Western medicine as our best chance for survival. We do not recommend abandoning traditional treatments such as surgery, radiation, and chemotherapy to pursue alternative therapies. Those of us who have experienced recurrence and/or metastasis are more willing to explore alternative therapies, but always as ancillary treatment in conjunction with traditional therapy. Some of the alternative therapies we have tried include acupuncture, massage, meditation, visualization, biofeedback, psychotherapy, diet modification, and non-FDA-approved therapeutics.

Donna relates, "I didn't look into any alternative therapies the first time I was diagnosed with breast cancer. But now that my tumor has metastasized, I'm pursuing some alternative therapies in conjunction with my regular medical care. If you had asked me two years ago if I thought I'd ever get into crystals, I wouldn't have even known what 'getting into crystals' meant. Now I wear a quartz crystal because a friend said it may enhance my immune

Today up to 50 percent of all cancer patients will seek complementary or alternative treatments in conjunction with traditional Western medical care. Contrary to popular opinion, the majority of these patients are well educated, at the early stage of disease, upper middle class, and are very knowledgeable about their disease.

The most common types of complementary therapy are diet changes, visualization, acupuncture, herbal remedies, and support groups.

Not only are many oncologists aware of these alternatives, many are recommending some of them to their patients.

Cassileth, B. R. "Unorthodox Cancer Medicine." *Cancer Investigation.* 4(6) (1986):591–98.

system. I still look at this disease from an intellectual perspective and still utilize Western medicine, and yet I don't think it hurts me a bit to look at other options."

Sally says, "I told my physician I wanted to take shark cartilage along with my chemotherapy. My physician said, 'Fine.' It's too soon to know if it really works—the research is still being conducted. It may turn out that I'm putting my money in a lot of different people's pockets for nothing. On the other hand, I can't be sure that the shark cartilage isn't at least part of the reason that my cancer didn't progress at all for a year and a half."

All of us have made changes in our diet and exercise habits in order to promote health and well-being. We believe that some complementary therapies may be useful as adjuncts to traditional treatments. But there are only so many hours in the day, especially when our jobs demand so much of our time. It has been difficult to find time for conventional therapy, let alone complementary treatments. Donna says, "It's important to live your life rather than living your cancer." We all agree.

We encourage:

- the use of traditional Western medicine
- complementary therapies to enhance your overall approach to your disease, and possibly improve your prognosis
- the realization that all treatment is time-consuming and physically, emotionally, and mentally taxing
- careful selection of complementary therapies that contribute to your overall well-being without excessive personal and professional trade-offs
- accepting your decision without regret, once it is made, while continuing to explore new options that may enhance your chances for cure

4

Experiencing Treatment

"I was mad. I thought, 'This is a hell of an inconvenience. This is screwing up my schedule.' I just didn't have time for it."

—*Joy Edwards*

Finding Time to Have Cancer

We have always recognized the need to balance the responsibilities of our personal and professional lives. We have each made a serious commitment to our career and are accustomed to working long hours yet still finding time for our friends and families. We know how to allocate our time effectively in order to fit all we can into each day's schedule.

When we were diagnosed with breast cancer, we faced a new and unexpected challenge: how to find time to gather information, to choose a course of action, to undergo treatment, and, at the same time, to care for ourselves. We discovered that, in addition to other physical and emotional ramifications, having breast cancer is extremely time-consuming.

Most of us were aware of the treatments for breast cancer: surgery, radiation, and chemotherapy. For those of us
who have made a major commitment to a career, anticipation of the disruptions caused by these therapies figured
largely in our initial reaction and approach to the disease.

A diagnosis of breast cancer means:

- significant disruption in work and personal
  schedules
- quickly learning new jargon and new
  environments
- developing new schedules for work and home
- learning to cope with stress precipitated by the
  potential loss of life versus normal stress from
  work and family

Our attitudes toward time, and the value we place on
it, have shaped our experiences with breast cancer. We
knew this disease would be a major disruption in our
schedules—and possibly a threat to our careers. The
prospect of adding another "responsibility" to our daily
activities was, and is, a disturbing thought—and more
than just a nuisance.

We find that we vary in the amount of attention we pay
to our health. While some of us consistently have annual
checkups, others do not.

We discovered the lumps in our breasts ourselves
through self-examination or through screening. Of those
of us who immediately sought medical advice, some were
told merely to monitor the lump over time. Joy did not
immediately seek medical help—she simply did not have
enough time. She knew it was going to be a serious problem but, at the time, felt that there were other life issues

A recent OSHA study to identify occupation as a risk factor for breast cancer mortality determined that managerial, clerical, and professional women faced increased risk of developing and dying from breast cancer. The mortality ratios for both Caucasian and African-American professionals were significantly higher than for nonprofessionals. Occupations at high risk for females include teachers, clergy, and librarians. The researchers were unable to find any predisposing workplace exposure that would explain the increased risk. The study cited many factors that may contribute to this increase in mortality risk, many of which are lifestyle choices such as age of the woman at first birth, choosing not to give birth and contraceptive use, although no conclusive evidence was cited. The study used a database of 2.9 million occupationally coded death certificates collected from twenty-three states from 1979 to 1987.

Hogfoss-Rubin, S., Burnett, C. C., Halperin, W. E., et al. "Occupation as a Risk Identifier for Breast Cancer." *American Journal of Public Health.* 83(9) (1993):1311–15.

that had to take priority. She was managing a very busy real estate business, raising teenaged children, and taking care of a medically disabled husband. Once her husband was able to return to work, she immediately sought medical attention. For all of us, our first thought was, I don't have time for this right now!—and this meant we had time neither to worry about it nor to fit medical appointments into our schedules. Most of all, we absolutely knew we couldn't take time out for surgery and treatment if it actually was breast cancer.

Even Daria, the physician in our group, found it difficult to schedule time to follow up. "When I found the lump, I went in for a mammogram, but it showed no change over the previous one, taken five years earlier, and the radiologist recommended waiting another year before having another one. So I decided to sit on the situation. Now I wish I'd had the lump removed right then. But I couldn't take time off work. When you run the entire operation, you can't call in sick without major consequences. There's no one standing by who can pick up the slack and cover for you."

Trade-Offs and Job Responsibilities

We assessed our responsibilities and immediately began planning ways to adjust our workload. In most cases, the reworking of our schedules not only allowed us to fit treatments into our daily routines, but it also enabled us to weather the treatments in what we term "a productive and effective manner."

Making it work at work:
- reorganize your responsibilities and routines to make sure all bases are covered
- adjust your schedule to include your treatment time
- look at your schedule adjustment as an opportunity
- decide if and how much time you can devote to your work
- expect to make some trade-offs
- expect to feel a sense of urgency about your work
- but, don't worry too much about your performance at work because your major concern should be your health

Each of us continued to work during therapy, scheduling our treatments in a way that minimized disruptions in our work. When necessary, we delegated or relinquished professional responsibilities, and some of us changed the nature of our jobs, either temporarily or permanently. We found ways to compensate for the times when we had to miss work or when we felt that our performance or productivity might be adversely affected by our treatment.

We each developed our own strategy for making it work at work. Daria wrote herself out of the daily patient care schedule and instead increased her administrative responsibilities. Betsy found that having her own law practice allowed her to pursue some new areas of law that had interested her for a long time. The move away from day-to-day management activities gave her time to take on breast cancer advocacy work and even focus on health and environmental law. She allocated some of her caseload to other attorneys, relinquished control or responsibility for other work, and refused to accept any new cases. After a sick leave from the university, Carol S. arranged to take a research leave to work on a project and had sufficient grant money to hire research assistants. Sally kept up with her teaching but practically abandoned her research and writing during this time. Cathy integrated the process in her day-to-day activities by using audiotaping, videotaping, and journaling for use in her television work. Joy cut her annual sales goals and hired assistants to work with her.

We all found that these adjustments have had some positive impact in our lives in one way or another. Daria felt she had never been able to get enough sleep—maybe three or four hours a night—and she was always tired. Because she increased her administrative work but eliminated patient care for five months (the time for surgery, chemotherapy, and a month to rebuild her white cell count and strengthen her immune system), she actually caught up on her sleep. "During those months, the emergency room ran more smoothly because I was able to catch up on the administrative side of our business. The staff liked to have me immediately available. So my being away from patient care had its good side."

Cathy believes that she was more productive at work during the months she was being treated for her recurrence of breast cancer. "I was thinking more clearly than ever before, and I had a mission. As we worked on the [television] documentary about my breast cancer, I assumed much more responsibility than ever before. Almost every day of those three months I marched in and said, 'Here's something for the series. Here's something we have to include.'"

In retrospect, most of us do not believe that our work performance was seriously compromised during our treatment, even though we had to significantly cut back on our activities.

Nonetheless, we did worry that our work was suffering. Concern about our ability to perform in our jobs was new to us. We were accustomed to feeling confident about our skills and abilities and in full control of our performance. Because a significant amount of our self-esteem is invested in our professional accomplishments and reputations, it was unsettling for us to suddenly feel insecure and anxious about our ability to perform. Cathy still receives calls every week from newly diagnosed women, and she tries to help them understand that "this is not the time to be superwoman. Trying to do too much right now can affect your healing." She reminds them that "cancer's a lousy hand to be dealt, but in the end we're all terminal . . . your last words on this earth are not going to be 'Gee, I wish I had spent more time in the office.'"

It is, of course, unrealistic to believe that the time commitment necessary for treatment, and our physical status during treatment, did not have an effect on our careers, or at least on our personal expectations of our careers. After all, most of us believe that no one can do our jobs better than we can. There were problems, and we made mistakes. We had to accept that patient care might suffer, a large contract might be lost, or important clients might be neglected. We found we had to do a lot more "clean-up and maintenance."

When we began to rearrange our lives to accommodate our treatment schedules, we found that the very skills that had brought us to this point in our careers were those we would and will continue to use.

Things to do for yourself:

- believe that this is your life, your time to concentrate on yourself
- acknowledge that there is time for therapy, for treatments
- structure your life carefully during these months
- be prepared to feel tired, sick, and less mentally sharp
- accommodate your physical and mental state—adjust
- put out fires
- delegate
- look forward to the time when your energy and vitality will return to their peak

Our sense of urgency and our commitment to our work actually helped us, giving us a focus—outside of our cancer and outside of ourselves—during the treatment phase. It helped us to realize that cancer was only one part of our lives. Donna reflects that "one of the things that got me through adjuvant chemotherapy was my work. I had

According to a publication by cancer survivors, employment can be a stabilizing influence for cancer survivors during a turbulent period. Work can be an opportunity to focus on something other than the illness and to be something more than a person with a disease. No studies have been done, to date, to evaluate whether survival is extended in people who continue to work.

Mullan, F., Hoffman, B. *Charting the Journey, An Almanac of Practical Resources.* Consumer Reports Books. Mt. Vernon, New York. 1990.

my treatments on Monday, and I always came back to work on Thursday or Friday, even though I didn't feel great. . . . My job forced me to focus on something else besides cancer. It reminded me that I had an identity separate from being a cancer patient." Carol S. found that sometimes "I was so absorbed with whatever I was doing that I hadn't thought to check my calendar for the next day [for treatment appointment]. It's extremely motivating to have a passion for your work, to have a focus outside of yourself."

The Experience of Surgery

Our reactions to hearing that we needed surgery ranged from panic to resignation. One of us was "absolutely terrified about what was happening" and thought there should be "some kind of manual or information about what will happen—how long you wait in preop, how cold the room is, why there are so many people around (and then no one)." She could have used detailed information on the experience from the patient's point of view. On the other hand Joy, who had been through so many surgeries, did not fear it but was decisive in what she wanted done—she had the experience and knew what was best for her. As Joy relates, "I chose to go in, have a frozen biopsy, and have the surgery at the same time. I have a rough time dealing with anesthetics, and that was the fifth or sixth surgery I'd had, so it wasn't something that I was looking forward to. I was more willing to have them make the choice than to go through being put under and coming back."

Surgery:

- comes at probably your most vulnerable time, usually right after diagnosis
- is easier to understand than other types of treatment
- causes emotional distress that usually passes quickly—probably because there are other important decisions to be made

Looking back, most of us don't view our surgery as being overly significant. Cathy says, "I wasn't away from the office very long for either my lumpectomy or my mastectomy, and both times I worked from the hospital. . . . The second time around, preparing for surgery (second opinions, etc.) actually kept me away from work more than the surgery itself. That time, I actually scheduled a personal retreat in the desert, four or five days prior to my operation, solely to meditate and pray about the surgery I was facing." We all believe, however, that the decision to have surgery came at a time when we were the most vulnerable—right after diagnosis—and that surgery was a contributing factor to our distress at that time.

> A study designed to assess the coping styles and stress levels of 117 women referred for breast biopsy determined that distress and perceived threat were greatest shortly after diagnosis. After surgery, patients' tension and stress level returned to prebiopsy level. For breast cancer patients, biopsy, diagnosis, and surgery tend to occur in rapid sequence so it is difficult to separate post-biopsy distress from distress engendered by the upcoming surgery.
>
> Stanton, A. L., Snider, P. R. "Coping with a Breast Cancer Diagnosis: A Prospective Study." *Health Psychology.* 12(1) (1993): 16–23.

We could argue that surgery is the one step we took that had a beginning, middle, and end—all within a relatively short time. It had the "closure" that was very important to us. Surgery isn't the unknown that radiation, chemotherapy, and the disease itself are. Because surgery removes the tumor, which is the root of our anxiety, the surgical process and its intended result are more tangible than radiation or chemotherapy. Surgery may, in fact, cause less stress than other therapies. Cathy says, "My attitude was, 'I'm really not sick, I felt fine before I came in here [the hospital].' I didn't allow surgery to stop me."

As noted earlier, reconstruction was viewed by Cathy and Daria as a positive aspect of their surgery. Because Cathy had previously had radiation, for the three weeks prior to her mastectomy, she applied vitamin E oil every night to the breast that would be removed. She also followed a regular regimen of vitamins, figuring that if she saturated her breast from the inside and out with vitamin E, it might make the skin heal faster and with less scarring. This routine was of her own invention, and she followed it because she was concerned about the pliability of her skin due to the radiation treatments after her lumpectomy three years earlier. Her surgeons had told her that radiation therapy probably would change the texture and resilience of the affected skin.

The tissue expansion process in reconstruction is a fairly simple procedure, and Cathy did not find it to be painful. But she experienced "a strange, almost claustrophobic feeling to have this foreign device within my now quite numb breast, which was being inflated to abnormal size and tightness. . . . I was still getting used to the loss of sensation and the strange new feeling of having a nonorganic thing under my skin." The expansion process went by quickly for Cathy. As mentioned earlier, she selected a silicone gel–filled implant with a textured silicone shell on the exterior.

Cathy's surgeries took place prior to the FDA's banning of the silicon implants in 1992 (except for women involved in long-range studies). She is still strongly in favor of implants, however. "I feel that the media and other public forums have done a great disservice to women by dividing us, as if the implant controversy is a sporting event on which we are expected to take sides and see who comes out the winner. This has been excruciating for those of us who are torn between our hope that we have triumphed over a terrible disease and the agony we feel for the small number who are experiencing problems that they believe were caused by these devices. I am concerned that the high level of anxiety will result in breast implants becoming unavailable in the near future, leaving women with fewer reconstructive options, and/or discouraging the research required to provide concrete answers to our questions about breast implants. Through all of this, I continue

In a study of sixty-three women receiving either immediate or delayed reconstruction the women receiving immediate reconstruction reported less difference in feelings of attractiveness and femininity as well as a notable absence of feelings of mutilation expressed by the delayed reconstruction group. Women who undergo immediate reconstruction tend to incorporate the new breast into their body image and therefore report a higher level of satisfaction in many areas, including sexuality.

The relationship between timing of reconstruction and the mastectomy experience also revealed a significant difference in distress levels. While only 25 percent of the women undergoing immediate reconstruction reported high levels of distress over mastectomy, 60 percent of the women opting for delayed reconstruction reported severe stress.

Both groups reported high satisfaction levels with their new breasts, with lack of sensation being the most frequently reported problem. The immediate reconstruction group reported more arm problems than did the delayed reconstruction group. This is due to the effect of the single operation, which combines reconstruction with ablation and axillary dissection.

Although the end point for delayed and immediate reconstruction may be equal, reduction of psychological distress may be a major benefit of immediate reconstruction.

Wellisch, D. K., Schain, W. S., Noone, R. B., et al. "Psychosocial Correlates of Immediate versus Delayed Reconstruction of the Breast." *Plastic and Reconstructive Surgery.* 76(5) (1985):713–18.

to have confidence in my doctors and even in the company that manufactured the implant that has been in my body for almost five years. I've had no problems with my implant, nor do I expect to have problems. I am satisfied with my breast reconstruction and grateful to the technology that has provided a device which is largely responsible for my psychological triumph over a devastating disease."

Waiting to Hear About the Nodes

During surgery, lymph nodes are removed from the area around the breast and under the arm, and samples are sent to the lab to see if cancer cells have spread to the nodes. There is usually a wait for test results following surgery. This waiting time is often very tense; some of us even said it was our "worst time." Cancer cells in the lymph nodes typically signal a more serious prognosis and nearly always determine the type of adjuvant therapy. Today, even with lumpectomy and no node involvement, some physicians are recommending chemotherapy in addition to radiation. A few years ago, however, standard treatment in this case was radiation alone. Probably the best way to prepare for these results is to read about the implications of node involvement and to be prepared to ask the physician specific questions. We know there are no guarantees, but we still view node involvement as an "indicator."

Finding out about node involvement is:

• a milestone because it tends to be an indicator of prognosis and helps determine the course of adjuvant therapy

- one of the most trying times during the course of your diagnosis

Donna's primary diagnosis was a medium-size tumor with no node involvement. She had radiation and chemotherapy, just in case, but two and a half years later her cancer metastasized. "And then in April I was diagnosed with metastatic breast cancer. I have bone disease. . . . The primary diagnosis was very scary; this was different. I was angry more than scared. I can no longer hope for a 'cure.'" We realize that what has happened in Donna's case could happen to any of us. It has been integrated into the dichotomy of our hope and despair, our ups and downs, and our fears and faith.

The Experience of Radiation and Chemotherapy

Radiation was not really as physically troublesome as we expected. Most of us did not feel ill or have significant side effects other than fatigue, although a few of us experienced muscle stiffness in our backs and upper arms (which can be reduced fairly easily by doing simple arm exercises regularly). But thinking about being somewhere other than work every day for six weeks was overwhelming, even if the therapy itself takes only minutes. It was distressing to realize that the treatments had to be done every day, that we had to arrange time to get to the hospital and back, and that it was all so time-consuming. Of course, we managed to fit it into our daily routine. Most of us redefined our roles and responsibilities. For example, some of us used the treatment time to get away from the office—to take a brisk walk to and from the treatment facility—to get something positive out of the experience. For some of us, it was actually a psychologically healing experience because our radiation therapy team became like a family. For Carol W., "It was one of the most positive aspects of my breast cancer experience. The people on my radiation team were caring and compassionate. They became like a family to me. It was one time of the day when I could let down my defenses and allow someone to show concern for me and take care of me."

Radiation therapy:

- side effects may not be as significant as anticipated in many cases
- treatment schedules may seem very inconvenient but actually can usually be accommodated into daily activities
- entails growing fatigue for most recipients

The daily treatments served as nagging reminders of the disease and, ironically, were even more disturbing if we were weathering the treatments well. Because the routine interrupted our daily work schedule, it never allowed us to forget that we were cancer patients.

We scheduled our treatments for early in the morning, late in the afternoon, or during lunchtime. Carol H. says, "I scheduled my treatments for midday and then I returned to work and stayed until eight o'clock or nine or ten or however long it took to accomplish what I needed to do."

A number of us chose to have a radiation booster implant (an extra amount of radiation to the spot where the tumor was). Because the radioactive substance in the booster implant may transmit rays outside the body, we were isolated from contact and, as a result, were also isolated from the support we were accustomed to receiving from our families and friends. Cathy relates, "My radiologist left the decision of whether to have implasty [radiation booster] completely up to me. I knew the straws would leave little scars on my breast and I made the radiologist draw dots on me to show what it would look like. I didn't decide until the last day of my daily radiation that I was going to check into the hospital and do that darn boost thing. That was the toughest part of my therapy— being in the hospital and seeing all these straws sticking out of my breast, making me look like a porcupine. I remember thinking, What have I let them do to me? But I'm glad I did it . . . otherwise I'd be blaming myself now for not doing everything I could have to keep this thing from coming back."

Boosters are an option:

- interstitial, internal, or radiation boosters are often used for treatment of breast cancer. A small amount of encapsulated radioactive material is placed directly into or close to the affected area.
- internal radiation therapy usually requires a hospital stay of from one to seven days

Chemotherapy, on the other hand, was for most of us a more negative experience. Compared to radiation, it required more juggling of our work schedules and even changes in our responsibilities. The start of chemotherapy treatment seemed to be the point at which we were most harshly brought face-to-face with our disease. Daria describes walking into the oncology clinic for her first chemotherapy treatment: "I saw all those bald people sitting in the waiting room and it suddenly struck me that I was a cancer patient just like them . . . and when I started chemotherapy, with almost immediate side effects, I realized 'Holy God, I really am sick.'"

Chemotherapy:

- causes more debilitating side effects than does radiation, so incorporating the treatments into your work routine requires planning
- side effects are temporary
- causes fatigue, nausea, some mental fuzziness

All of us received our chemotherapy on an outpatient basis. Most of us struggled with chemotherapy's side effects, including nausea and vomiting, fatigue, hair loss, lack of energy, weight gain or loss, and difficulty concentrating. Donna was treated on Monday, was "doped up" at home until Tuesday, and was very sick for another day, then returned to work on Thursday and Friday. Sally scheduled her chemotherapy for Thursday afternoons after her last lecture, then vomited and slept through the weekend so she could drag herself back to work on Monday. Betsy says, "I was nauseated or felt like I had an upset stomach the entire time" and, as is fairly customary, ate to try to relieve the nausea. It didn't really help—she just gained weight.

Carol S. told us, "During treatment, each month became a kind of blur that I couldn't explain. My brain seemed absorbed, and it was hard work to reach it, to rope it in and put it to a task. Each day I would line up what I wanted to accomplish, write it down, and then cir-

Contrary to popular opinion, over 50 percent of all breast cancer patients experience a weight gain of six to fourteen pounds. At a time when self-image and self-esteem may be lower than normal, weight gain may be an additional stress. Researchers also fear that the increased weight may portend a poorer prognosis. Changes in metabolic rate, physical activity, and diet may all play a role in weight gain although no firm data exist to support any of these mechanisms. A pilot study has begun to determine which areas are in need of further research.

Stockwell, S. "Breast Cancer Weight Gain: New Research May Help Solve the Puzzle." *Oncology Times.* 15(9) (1993): 1–17.

cle slowly around the house like a cat looking for a place to have kittens. Within a couple of weeks after I completed chemo and radiation, I noticed that I was at my computer writing again, I was returning phone calls with some regularity, I cleaned out my closet, and I finished a paper that I had begun six months earlier. The files were dated in my computer suggesting that I had tried working on the same paper during chemo, but no progress was made. . . . Only in retrospect can I reflect on this and comprehend how very fuzzy my thinking was. . . . The chemistry of the brain must be very delicate. I feel clear-headed again [now that I am no longer on chemotherapy]. Nowhere did I read about this aspect of the treatment." The mental "fuzziness" was disturbing until we realized what was causing it—and that it would go away. These side effects and the amount of time chemotherapy required forced most of us to make significant changes in our work schedules, either temporarily or permanently.

Chemotherapeutic side effects, including nausea, hair loss, and exhaustion, are experienced by more than 80 percent of all cancer patients. The problems caused by the side effects of chemotherapy may become so severe that treatment may be discontinued. Studies have shown that at least 46 percent of cancer patients receiving chemotherapy have had thoughts about discontinuing treatment, but only a few discussed this with their medical team. By discussing their concerns regarding the side effects of chemotherapy with their oncology team, patients may be able to receive advice on how to manage the side effects of chemotherapy and may be more likely to continue treatment.

Love, R. R., Loventhal, H., Easterling, D. V., et al. "Side Effects and Emotional Distress during Cancer Chemotherapy." *Cancer.* 63 (1989):604–12.

The permanent changes we have made were by choice because we found they fit better with the way we now viewed our lives.

In the last few years, antinausea drugs have improved, and some of us believe they are a godsend. During Sally's first round of chemotherapy, the antinausea drug tended "to make her groggy." During her second round of chemotherapy, she took Zofran®, which she says "is a miracle drug." Zofran almost completely relieved her vomiting and nausea (and she was taking one of the heaviest doses of chemotherapy given). Daria, who was in a clinical trial and also receiving heavy doses of chemotherapy, also took an antinausea drug nearly the entire time, but she was still sick. She supposes it relieved the nausea somewhat, but "I couldn't imagine how I could have felt worse!"

In addition to nausea, chemotherapy may temporarily cause:

- changes in skin color—sallowness
- hair loss
- significant weight gain or loss

Of the six of us who had chemotherapy, three lost nearly all body hair and two had some hair loss or thinning. Joy feared losing her hair because of her need, as a realtor, to maintain her public image. Joy says, "I have to tell you, I had no hair on any part of my body, but my head and . . . I swear to this day I willed it to stay there, and it did. I'll never know why."

Some of us had a runny nose throughout the months of chemotherapy because there was no hair to catch nasal secretions. Daria relates, "I ran into an old friend . . . and he [asked], 'What's been going on?' I told him, 'I've had cancer and blah, blah,' and he said 'How was your runny nose?' I thought, How did you know about my runny nose? He said his grandfather had chemo and . . . lost all his hair and . . . he didn't have any nose hairs to hold it. I said, 'Oh my God, it's the nose hairs! There are no nose hairs to hold the normal secretions!' But you never hear that talked about."

We each attempted to keep a sense of humor about our hair loss. Both times Donna lost her hair, she shaved her head as soon as her hair started falling out. Sally says she looked forward to not having to shave her legs—there had to be something positive in the experience. However, as she explains, "I have no hair on my head, I have no hair under my arms, but I have the hairiest legs! I think God is playing a joke on me." And, Daria jokes, "When I was bald, my husband would breathe on my head and pretend to polish it. He called me 'CD' for chrome dome. Later he called me 'FD' for fuzz dome. You have to hang on to your sense of humor."

Not everyone experienced nausea and hair loss. For example, Carol S. felt fatigued but rarely had nausea. She attributes this, in part, to the way she planned her day after each treatment. Rather than going home or to bed, she went immediately for a walk at the ocean nearby in San Francisco to take in plenty of fresh air. In fact, the one time she drove directly home she got sick. She made the days of her treatments a special occasion. "I invited a friend to go with me on the days I went to the clinic for my chemotherapy. It was a chance to spend a day in San Francisco, something I don't do often enough because I always seem to be overscheduled. After my treatment, we would walk on the beach and treat ourselves to dinner at a great restaurant, then a double feature. I almost looked forward to those days. My friends wanted to be included in my schedule."

Maintaining a Work Persona

We did not want to appear sick or vulnerable to our colleagues, clients, students, and customers during our treatment. We realized physical appearance is an important part of our professional image or work persona, and we did our best to cope with changes in our physical appearance during the treatment phase. We felt that we were often on display because of our cancer, and we wanted to be perceived as strong and in control rather than as needing sympathy. Chemotherapy was responsible for most of the visible changes to our appearance, which included a sallow look to our skin, loss of hair, and weight gain or loss.

Maintaining at work while undergoing treatment:

- it may be difficult to maintain and manage to "look good"
- fatigue and general discomfort may make it difficult to keep emotions under control
- you can develop ways to work around these encumbrances
- you can choose whom, at work, you want to tell about your treatment

It is sometimes difficult to continue working during treatment—to continue functioning in a business or professional environment—because we know that some of our talent and success is attributed to our appearance or persona. A "bad hair day" or clothes that are too tight or too baggy can be depressing to the healthiest of us. Add to that extreme fatigue and the feeling of being "on display" because of our disease, and the result is something less than an emotional high.

We believed that it was important to "package" ourselves by wearing a wig or by applying extra makeup so that we looked as normal and healthy as possible. Many of us found we could take only so much sympathy, only so much "tiptoeing" around the subject, only so much "Gee, you look great." Some of us also felt a responsibility to try not to look normal all the time. As Carol S. says, "When I'd go into work to pick up my mail, people would say, 'You look fantastic. You look just wonderful. Can we have some of whatever you're taking?' It was hard for me to take on days when I was pale and didn't think I looked too great. Sometimes I thought I had a responsibility to look as bad as I felt. I wanted my appearance to say, 'This is cancer. This is serious.'"

With the exception of the initial diagnosis of cancer, loss of hair (alopecia) may be the most traumatic side effect that cancer patients will experience. Hair loss is, for many cancer patients, a constant reminder of their illness. A study of forty cancer patients demonstrated significant differences in body images between patients losing hair due to chemotherapy and patients not losing their hair. The researchers suggest the following for areas of further study: examining other side effects of chemotherapy on body image, and whether preparing a patient for loss of hair has any impact on body image.

Boxley, K. O., Erdman, L. K., Henry, E. B., et al. "Alopecia: Effect on Cancer Patients' Body Image." *Cancer Nursing.* 7(6) (1984):499–503.

In addition to coping with changes in our physical appearance, we had to deal with the reactions of our clients, customers, and coworkers as a result of their knowing that we were undergoing therapy for breast cancer. All of us have jobs that involve a great deal of responsibility, and we were concerned about the impact on our clients, customers, and organizations if we made mistakes. We took precautions. Betsy says, "Each time I was on chemotherapy, I experienced a slowing down of my ability to think and remember. My oncologist kept saying that there should not be a loss of cognitive abilities. However, I still felt that for a certain number of days after the actual chemotherapy treatment I had a hard time focusing, and I kept losing things, especially my reading glasses. During these periods, I made sure that my assistant reviewed anything of importance. I wanted to be sure I hadn't overlooked something or made a mistake.

Concentration was difficult. In retrospect, some of the perceived side effects could well have been the results of a drastic diminishment of estrogen and the trauma of a diagnosis of cancer. Many times I think we all underestimate the trauma of a diagnosis. I figured that my concentration would return and I simply had to compensate. For example, I went to the drugstore and bought ten pairs of reading glasses so that I could always lay my hands on at least one pair."

Joy lost two clients because they chose to find another realtor after hearing that she was having chemotherapy. As she says, "They thought I couldn't keep up with them . . . and they didn't want to wear me out. Following those experiences, I stopped telling clients about my cancer."

Betsy also found that she needed to be selective in disclosing her condition. She relates, "When clients call, they want you to be there to answer their questions or solve their problems. I didn't want them to think I would be unavailable for long periods of time. It doesn't sound

---

Many cancer survivors have found that co-workers, clients, and customers may hold misconceptions about the severity of cancer and cure rates. Many people will wonder if and when you are going to die, while others may be shocked that you look so healthy. Co-workers and clients may wonder if you are able to continue to carry out your job as effectively. These concerns may lead to covert discrimination and may limit the disclosure of information regarding cancer treatment by the cancer patient.

Mullan, F., Hoffman, B. *Charting the Journey, An Almanac of Practical Resources.* Consumer Reports Books. Mt. Vernon, New York. 1990.

good when your secretary says, 'Oh, she's out having chemotherapy today.' So my secretary and I worked out how she would answer the phone and what she would tell particular clients." We have all found ways to work around the demands and expectations of our work environment.

5

Fallout at Work

"You want to make sure that your performance [at work] is an Academy Award winner, and after you've performed you can go backstage and collapse and they can carry you out in an ambulance; but while you're onstage there's a certain persona you must exhibit."
—**Carol Washington**

The fact that we are breast cancer survivors affects both our current and potential future employment. We have all continued to work throughout our treatment for breast cancer, yet we are concerned about the long-term effects that being a cancer survivor will have on our professional lives.

Implications:
- insurance
- health
- disability
- life
- ability to transfer and/or change jobs
- earning ability
- long-term career goals

- reactions of colleagues
- credibility

Each of us reevaluated our jobs and the decisions we had made in the past about how we apportioned our time between professional and personal commitments and, more importantly, how we would now approach our professional commitments. Amy relates, "In the middle of a Tuesday afternoon, I was startled to find myself in a reverie about the meaning of life, examining my priorities, questioning if my work—fairly equivalent to my life—was making a difference to humankind. Does it really matter to the world if I do one more successful public offering, merger, or reorganization? Does it really matter to me?" And we have all begun the process of determining the professional roles we want to play in the future. Such introspection about one's professional life happens to most people at some point, but for us it was precipitated at an earlier time as a result of our diagnoses. In a way, breast cancer has accelerated our professional maturity. Many of the pursuits and areas of responsibility in which we might have invested time and energy prior to our diagnosis of breast cancer no longer seem so important. A number of us have integrated the issues involving our diagnosis of breast cancer into our work goals in creative ways. For example, Carol W. was already on the staff of Cancer Care, where a tremendous amount of breast cancer education takes place. Betsy and Sally are incorporating breast cancer work into their established positions. And Amy, as executive director of NABCO, has essentially made breast cancer her career.

We have found that both our employers' prejudices about cancer and the issues of health insurance and other benefits can have a direct impact on our ability to change careers or even to make career moves. We understand, from experience, that women who have survived breast cancer may be forced to base far-reaching career decisions on the continued availability of health insurance coverage rather than on considerations of professional or job satisfaction.

We feel it is important that every woman become familiar with the specifics of her disability and health insurance coverage. She should become aware of whether her insurance coverage can be carried to another job; her current and any possible future benefits packages and sick leave policies, including how any time spent on sick leave affects retirement; and her rights under the Americans with Disabilities Act of 1991 (ADA).

Health Insurance

Not only does having breast cancer disrupt your earnings, but the diagnostic and treatment phases are also very expensive. Even with insurance coverage, deductibles and noncovered expenses must be paid out-of-pocket. Experimental treatments may pose an even greater financial risk. Although Sally's insurance company did cover the cost of her stem-cell transplant, this type of coverage is not always available because many insurance policies do not reimburse for experimental treatments.

There are also unexpected costs indirectly caused by having cancer, for example, the need to hire an assistant, as did Carol S., or take on a partner, as did Joy, or costs associated with travel and housing when seeking care out of state. In addition, Carol S. had a nine-hundred-dollar telephone bill in the period following her diagnosis due to the number of calls she returned to colleagues, friends, and family.

Insurance issues are a major concern for anyone with cancer. Fortunately, most of us are covered by health insurance policies that provided sufficient coverage so that the financing of our treatment has not become an overwhelming burden. However, Joy's medical insurance, which she receives as part of her deceased husband's corporate retirement and death benefits, will expire soon. As she states, "If national health doesn't become a reality, I'll just have to die because I can't afford to stay alive."

Each state currently has a mechanism for providing health insurance for the uninsurable. However, the premiums are high and the coverage is not commensurate with the medical costs. Along with work-related health insurance also comes life insurance and, sometimes, disability insurance. An independent insurance plan is almost impossible to secure after a diagnosis of cancer. Some group plans do offer open enrollment but have exclusionary clauses that preclude benefits to someone with a progressive disease.

Employability and insurability are intertwined in our society because health insurance is normally provided as a benefit of employment. Cancer survivors may not be able to transport health insurance from one employer to another. Preexisting condition limitations may pose serious problems for cancer survivors by limiting coverage for certain conditions for a significant length of time or even for life.

Sick Leave

Our experiences with sick-leave policies were varied and were related to whether we work for others or are self-employed.

Carol S. found that her university offers its faculty an excellent sick-leave policy, which allowed her to take a semester off from teaching at full pay.

Sally is also a professor, but her experience with her university was less satisfactory. Sally remembers, "Before I knew that my cancer was going to progress and I would have a stem-cell transplant, I asked the university for a sabbatical leave. I had never asked for time off throughout the two years of surgery, radiation, metastasis, and chemotherapy. I had missed very few classes and had scheduled medical appointments and treatments around my teaching schedule. I had often taught while fuzzy headed and on antinausea drugs or painkillers. I wanted a year in which to put the cancer first, scheduling treatments when it was best to have them and staying in bed when I was sick or in pain. The state university system denied my request for sabbatical leave because I had only been in the Florida system for four years; the administration would not give me paid time off. If I couldn't teach my classes, I wouldn't get paid. Perhaps I didn't 'look' sick. I had made every effort to look normal by wearing a wig that closely matched my own hair. On my good days, and most were good days, I looked fine and was full of energy. On my really pain-filled days, I was at home in bed, full of morphine. I guess they couldn't relate—if I didn't act or look sick in front of them, even though they knew I was on chemotherapy, I must not be sick. I eventually successfully negotiated for half pay for research and administrative work, with no teaching. When it became certain that I would have the bone-marrow transplant, I was amazed to find out that the only paid leave I could get was the forty-four days of sick leave that I had earned over the four years I had been at the University. Five of the seven months I was away from work for the transplant and recovery were without pay. If I had not taken out a long-term disability policy on my own, I would be in serious financial trouble now."

Cathy has been the chief assistant to a very busy television executive for thirteen years and was concerned about what her recovery time would mean to him. She made sure that when she did return to work, she was able to do so with full faculties and energy, comparable to her abilities before her surgery. She worries about what might have happened or will happen if she needs chemotherapy. "Perhaps I would have offered to step down from my position. This would have been difficult for me because I really love my job. I still worry at times about this happening to me in the future. I've had one recurrence already. What if it comes back? Will it cost me my job?"

Like many women who are self-employed or work as independent contractors, Joy works on commission. She does not have paid sick leave and, in fact, has no income if she fails to produce sales every day.

Disability Insurance

Some of us have excellent short- and long-term disability coverage provided by our employers, and others of us have purchased such policies on our own. For example, Daria had her own policy, which began payments after a three-month waiting period. We have found that most disability policies have specific exclusionary clauses and significant waiting periods, so it is fairly common to have to draw on savings or other resources until the waiting period expires. Carol S. was able to go on the state disability program but was almost excluded from that resource due to an administrative error. Because of her medical history, Joy has been unable to obtain any type of insurance protection for lost work time for the past twenty-five years.

Americans with Disabilities Act

Though breast cancer survivors are legally considered "disabled" as defined by the Americans with Disabilities Act (ADA), as a group, we do not consider ourselves to be disabled. We recognize the stigma attached to this label and emphasize that disability from breast cancer does not influence our abilities to function effectively in our jobs. (Although some of us did note that chemotherapy seemed to have negative effects on our ability to concentrate and solve problems with our usual acuity, that could also have resulted from the high level of stress we each felt during treatment.) We are aware that many cancer survivors are perceived to be handicapped and, as a result, may face repercussions at work. Approximately one-fourth of cancer survivors have experienced some form of employment discrimination based on their medical history alone. While the ADA affords some protection for cancer survivors, primarily as a deterrent to employers, we know that discrimination against women who have survived breast cancer, or any other kind of cancer, has not been eliminated.

The Americans with Disabilities Act, a federal civil rights law, says that prospective employers cannot ask about a person's medical history or current medical conditions. The ADA also says that employees cannot be demoted or fired because of a disability if the person is oth-

The work-related problems of the over five million cancer survivors may encompass many areas. Dismissal, failure to hire or promote, demotion, denial of benefits, and hostility of co-workers are examples of both covert and overt discrimination.

Hoffman, B. "Cancer Survivors at Work: Job Problems and Illegal Discrimination." *Oncology Nursing Forum.* 16(1) (1989):39–42.

erwise able and qualified to do the job (cancer is considered a disability under this Act). Despite this law, cancer-based discrimination, either subtle or blatant, does occur, and can include not being hired in the first place, being passed over for promotions, demoted, transferred to an undesirable position, or even fired.

Carol H. joined a major corporation in 1978 as a sales representative in the field and worked her way to an executive position at corporate headquarters. Shortly after she finished treatment in 1989, she was asked to step down from her position because top management was concerned about her health. Carol says, "I was stunned and angry. I hadn't taken a day off during my treatment or ever used my illness as an excuse. I had juggled my schedules for treatment, my work, and being a single mother of two boys." She is no longer with that company.

In 1990, Joy was fired in spite of the fact that she was one of the top producing agents for her real estate company. She was so outraged that she sued the company for breach of contract and discrimination against the handicapped. The jury awarded her nearly half a million dollars in general and punitive damages. Joy relates, "I think the company fired me in part because I wanted to cut

The following are some suggestions for dealing with on-the-job discrimination:

- If you feel that you are being discriminated against due to your medical history, let your employer know that you are aware of your legal rights. Tactfully convey the message that you would rather work out an informal arrangement than resort to the legal system for protection.
- Be aware of antidiscrimination filing dates. Many states have 180-day filing periods for antidiscrimination complaints; after this deadline it is very difficult to file a complaint.
- If you need to adjust your work schedule (flextime or leave of absence), provide your employer with alternatives.
- Educate your employer and co-workers about the survival rates for your specific type of cancer.
- Seek the support of co-workers. They have a vested interest in protecting themselves from discrimination.
- Keep accurate written records of all job actions both positive and negative. Include performance evaluations that demonstrate your abilities. Also include any negative actions taken by your employer that may be the result of your cancer diagnosis. These will be helpful if you have to go to court.
- Use community resources and support groups.
- Be prepared to face the results of your decision to fight. Positive outcomes may include continued employment and/or insurance benefits, monetary gain, and a personal sense of justice. Negative results may include a long legal battle, stress, and a negative relationship with the people you sue.

Mullan, F., Hoffman, B. *Charting the Journey, An Almanac of Practical Resources for Cancer Survivors.* Consumer Reports Books. Mt. Vernon, New York. 1990.

back on my rigorous work pace. Even at a reduced pace, I was selling more than three million dollars' worth per year. And I had worked for the company and its predecessor for more than twenty years." Her legal case was settled in 1990. Joy has moved to another agency, where she is one of the top producers. She feels that had she not fought this unfair action she would not be alive today because she would have allowed herself to accept the victim's position.

Life Insurance

Obtaining life insurance can also be a problem. It is now almost impossible for some of us to add to our existing policies, which makes it more difficult for us to leave a legacy to our children or grandchildren. There is a "guaranteed issue" policy for which no physical exam is required and no medical questions asked on the simple one-page application. However, the cost is high and benefits are accrued over time, meaning that benefits are reduced if death occurs within the first few years after purchase of the policy.

Those of us who have good policies feel lucky; we have done our part to ensure that those we love will not face financial hardships. But, in a way, our need to keep our families financially secure constrains our own choices, especially regarding our freedom to engineer our own deaths if, because of disease progression, we should choose to do so. Life insurance policies usually do not insure for suicide, and those of us who would like to have that option must carefully assess the ramifications.

Changing Jobs

The degree of "entrenchment" in one organization may compromise our ability to change jobs, especially if the new position requires full disclosure about our medical condition. Changing jobs, like securing health insurance, can be almost impossible after the diagnosis of cancer. Many women find themselves forced to remain in positions that have become unsatisfactory because of co-workers' attitudes, job-related stress, suspected discrimination, or being passed up for promotions simply because they have cancer.

While we may feel secure in our present work situations, we are uncertain about what would happen if we were to change employers or careers. For example, we may choose to change, or be forced to change, careers or working arrangements as we reorder our priorities and how we spend our time. Betsy believes that her age and history of breast cancer make it unlikely that any law firm would hire her. Daria acknowledges that her ability

---

Many breast cancer survivors perceive limited marketability and freedom in changing employers, a phenomenon referred to as "job lock." This phenomenon occurs when a woman or her partner is afraid to change jobs for fear of losing benefits such as health, disability, and life insurance coverage.

American Society of Clinical Oncology Committee on Patient Advocacy. "The Physician as the Patient's Advocate" (editorial). *Journal of Clinical Oncology.* 11(6) (1993):1011–13.

Tips for avoiding work-related discrimination:

- Do not volunteer information about cancer survivorship. Unless your medical history directly affects your ability to perform your job, you have no obligation to disclose this information.
- Be truthful when filling out employment applications. Dishonesty may be grounds for termination of work and/or insurance benefits.
- Apply for jobs for which you are qualified.
- Lessen the impact of a gap in employment (caused by treatment, recovery, termination of employment due to illness, etc.) by organizing your résumé topically instead of chronologically.
- If you have to explain a gap in employment convey that your illness is in the past and that you are in good health and expect to remain in good health.
- Seek the help of a career counselor. A professional will help you formulate honest answers for interview questions that may be difficult.
- Seek employers who are federally prohibited from disability discrimination. For example, federal departments and agencies are required to have affirmative action policies and are therefore less likely to discriminate.
- Do not think of yourself as handicapped. Assess your strengths and go after jobs that fit your needs.

Mullan, F., Hoffman, B. *Charting the Journey, An Almanac of Practical Resources for Cancer Survivors.* Consumer Reports Books. Mt. Vernon, New York. 1990.

to leave her current environment for another practice in another state is unlikely, if the position were to include management responsibilities. And those working in small businesses or for nonprofit organizations are also severely limited in their ability to change jobs. Because of the prohibitive cost of insurance, these organizations—unjustly but supposedly out of necessity—will frequently choose a candidate who has a clean bill of health over one who has a chronic and possibly terminal disease.

On the Job

Being a survivor of breast cancer may also affect the level of income and career moves available to you in the years ahead. We believe that our diagnoses will have an effect on our professional "progression." We have evaluated our career plans and our professional goals and have had to come to terms with alternatives we believe will be as rewarding, but perhaps less taxing than our work before our diagnoses (especially for those of us with metastatic disease). Our financial security may be affected by career changes, and, of course, this is a major consideration for us. But we have found it more difficult to readjust our thinking about our careers. The concept of career carries with it a significant number of intangibles: feelings of accomplishment and competence, feelings of worth and value, recognition, confidence and control, respect, challenge and excitement. Most of us feel that our careers provide us with much of our identities. These issues have, as a result, been more difficult to "rework" than the financial issues.

Metropolitan Life Insurance Company and the now defunct Bell Telephone Company conducted studies of their employees with a history of cancer to determine the effects of chronic illness on productivity. Both studies concluded that there was little difference between cancer survivors and other employees in regard to turnover, absence, and work performance. Both companies concluded that hiring cancer survivors was a sound industrial practice.

Hoffman, B. "Cancer Survivors at Work: Job Problems and Illegal Discrimination." *Oncology Nursing Forum.* 16(1) (1989): 39–43.

Things to consider about relationships with others:

- your own need for privacy
- the strain of dealing with others' distress about your illness
- the effect of your diagnosis on how others perceive you in the workplace
- how having the spotlight on you fits with your responsibility as a role model for colleagues, subordinates, and students
- your personal philosophy and mission

Donna says about leaving her job that "I want to time when I go out on sick leave perfectly. I want to do a brilliant transition memo for my successor, clean out my desk, and walk out with my head high. But deciding which time is right is very tough. I don't want the memory I leave to be that of an ineffective, bald person who shuffles out the door."

Reactions of Colleagues

Because of cancer phobia, the work environment to which the breast cancer survivor returns may be hostile, and she may be afraid to discuss the situation with her manager for fear of retribution. Management itself may harass the employee in an attempt to provoke her resignation. The company Joy worked for harassed her for two years by, among other things, taking away her reserved parking space and asking that she share an office (moves that were viewed as demotions) before firing her.

A diagnosis of cancer has other work-related ramifications, including the reactions of our colleagues and our credibility with them. The one thing none of us wanted was for our colleagues to be openly sympathetic, as this stripped away our veneer of coping and our strength. We could cry in private or with family members or close friends, but our public persona needed to be left intact. Joy used a signal when she arrived at the office by saying it was a one- or two-hug day. Others of us avoided people we knew would tear up as they told us how sorry they were. Humor was welcome, as were people who could help us express our anger and frustration.

However, many of our relationships at work did change. We made new friends when people, who had secret histories of cancer themselves or in their families, came out of the closet. We all began to serve as role models for dealing with breast cancer. Some of us did not have to worry about what our diagnosis meant in terms of our credibility because, as Daria states, "It really depends on how well seated you are in your establishment." The longer a person has been around, the more likely it is she

will garner a lot of support. But others of us felt we lost
credibility, or at least felt that management did not believe we would have the strength and fortitude to handle
any assignment, no matter what the demands. Otherwise,
why would Carol H. have been asked to assume another
position? And, in fact, one of us was asked to select her
professional successor.

Problems related to workplace attitudes:

- ostracism by colleagues, superiors, subordinates
- overt hostility from colleagues
- complaints from colleagues about leaning too
  much on others
- inability to cope with overly solicitous or
  protective behavior
- implications from colleagues that the cancer
  survivor is no longer capable of self-management

Managing Relationships with Others

The more we were able to dictate the degree of others' information and participation, the greater our sense of privacy and control. Most of us found ways to withhold the
news about our diagnosis until we felt comfortable releasing it, and then we decided whom to tell and how. After sharing the news with our immediate circle of family
and friends, we had to decide who else should be told.

In addition to our concerns regarding privacy, the decision of whom in our work environments we told about
our diagnosis involved issues of visibility, vulnerability,
and pride in productivity. Some of us were concerned

about our ability to maintain our composure when discussing our diagnoses with colleagues and subordinates. Others of us felt that knowledge of our disease might have negative consequences in the workplace—peers, subordinates, or organizations might discriminate against us in terms of future work assignments and promotions. And, indeed, some of us eventually did experience discrimination at work because of our breast cancer. Amy suffered a different kind of discrimination. As she relates, "One night, at about 9:00 P.M., I was working in my office, with one hand on the calculator and the other holding an ice pack to my chest, which was becoming a little swollen and uncomfortable from the radiation. A number of the firm's managing directors had passed my office earlier in the evening, headed to the executive dining room to celebrate the closing of a major transaction. The dinner over, they were strolling out, one by one, in a cloud of cigar smoke, cheered by good cognac and the prospect of high fees. One of the firm's partners passed my open door, stopped, came back, and leaning against the door frame, said reflectively, 'You know, you've always had great tits. So with one great tit, you're still in better shape than a lot of women.' 'Get out of my office,' I said and, in two strides, closed the door. Despite the big money and title, I knew it was definitely time to change jobs."

A few of us chose to tell only one or two close friends at work. Others expanded the network of those who knew, and Cathy even went nationwide with the news.

Carol W. relates, "I finally decided not to burden the support staff at the office with the facts of my situation. That worked very well for me. Over time, I began to share with selected other people at work. I told people on my own terms, and that made me feel more in control of the situation."

However, Carol S. says, "I didn't feel it was right to simply disappear and have a parade of graduate students teach my classes and tell my students that I was off on a trip. My students are mostly young women, and I wanted them to hear the news directly from me. I hated for them to hear in another way, or worse, for one of them someday to find a lump in her breast and be too afraid to do anything about it. And being honest with my students made me feel a little bit innovative. Each of us has figured out a more courageous way to share the news because of the people who have come before us. I wanted to be a role model for my students and for the other faculty women who would be diagnosed after me."

Cathy chose to tell not only the people she worked with about her recurrence of breast cancer, but also to inform millions of women across the country by doing a television documentary about her situation. She explains, "Just a few days before my mastectomy, a friend suggested that I consider documenting my experience in some way. This had never occurred to me, and my first reaction was to decline. This was back in 1989, and as yet no network television program had attempted to follow a woman through breast cancer surgery and treatments. My boss thought I was crazy to want to put myself through that when I was about to have a mastectomy, but I felt strongly that doing the show could help women by increasing their awareness of, and knowledge about, breast cancer. I am a Christian, and I thought God was challenging me to share this part of my life with others. Maybe that was part of the reason why I had breast cancer. . . . I felt very uncomfortable telling the whole country that I was losing my breast. But I know it helped a lot of women, and I'm glad I did it."

Strength and Vulnerability

We find that vulnerability is not acceptable, except in those rare situations when it works to a woman's advantage to put on the "human" mantle. Many of us equate vulnerability with weakness, not necessarily because it is our personal belief, but rather because we have seen rewards given to the strong and penalties handed to the weak. Irrespective of personal belief, the work environment tends to dictate professional behavior. While we are not averse to using manipulation to achieve our objectives, we are typically loath to use what is perceived as female "weaknesses" to get our desired results. We value resilience more highly than bravado. In fact, it is probably true that we push ourselves harder to weather major disturbances with finesse and style. And therein often lie the personal and professional rewards.

Some strategies to keep emotions in check at work:

- tell people directly that sympathy does not always help
- have a colleague or spouse run "interference"
- establish "signals" with coworkers so they know when to ask questions
- set limits on the number of social contacts you have during your business day
- cry when you're at home
- when angry, use a pillow to beat against your bed or a wall, or find a private place outdoors where you can rage as loud and long as you need to

There is a feeling among us of having a role to play—of being on display and having no choice in the matter. But as Carol W. says, "It's your own self-esteem. It's your own self-image, and you're not going to let anything get in the way of making sure that your performance [at work] is an Academy Award winner. After you've performed you can go backstage and collapse and they can carry you out in an ambulance, but while you're onstage there's a certain persona you must exhibit."

In one situation, Betsy had to request a continuance for a trial scheduled for the week following her chemotherapy treatment. She said the other lawyers and the judge were very understanding, but she hated the fact that she "had to tell them why I needed a continuance for that particular week. I felt as if the attorney from the other side was thinking, 'Ah, she's going through chemotherapy. . . . Maybe I have an advantage over her. . . . Maybe she won't be as sharp as she usually is.' I believe many attorneys would think that, whether they're proud of it or not. It bothered me. I didn't want to appear weak or vulnerable."

We have spoken with a number of professional women who have refused to discuss their breast cancer in public. Many women will talk with someone one-on-one or will offer information anonymously. But there seems to be a belief that "going public" is too much of a risk for most of us. Cathy went public by appearing on national television, Amy went public when she assumed the directorship of NABCO and a position on the board of the National Breast Cancer Coalition, and Betsy has gone public by serving on the board of directors of the National Breast Cancer Coalition. And every year, during Breast Cancer Awareness Month, Joy gives a presentation on breast cancer to the hundreds of realtors in her company.

As professional women, we have all had to sacrifice something to get where we are. We wanted a career more than we wanted a traditional kind of life, especially those of us who made that decision during the years when it was not a comfortable choice. For Betsy, going to law school "at the time I did and getting established in my profession in the 1970s was a struggle. None of the men said, 'Hey great, here's Betsy, come on in.' I had to struggle for professional respect and recognition. And I don't want to risk my credibility now by appearing vulnerable."

We did not want to bring our feelings, especially strong emotions, to the workplace. As Betsy says, "It is absolutely imperative, and it's always been a part of the rules of the game and part of a profession—you never cry . . . it's just a rule. Whether that's right or wrong, that's the way [it is]—it's like you're a joke. The minute you cry, whether it's appropriate or not . . . it's not acceptable in any circumstance. . . . That rule was and still exists today: You're in a professional setting—a 'warrior mode'—and you can't cry. You totally destroy yourself as a professional. Then someone says, 'She can't handle it.'"

Daria feels, "I don't want to cry in front of the people I work with because I know they are looking at me as a role model, and they're watching closely to see how I'm handling breast cancer. I want to be an exemplary role model. I want to be the epitome of strength, decisiveness, and caring. Being strong is a critical piece of the way I see myself as a professional woman and a critical piece of the way others see me. People look at me and say, 'How the hell did you do what you've done? You're an inspiration to us because you got back into the ring.' And that's what I want to hear."

Being emotional is taxing; but we have all learned that controlling our emotions also takes energy. It was not unnatural or unusual for us to want to cry, especially when a particularly close or sympathetic colleague approached us with concern. Nor was it unusual to feel less able to control these feelings when we were physically and emotionally weak from treatment and its side effects. For Daria it meant telling coworkers, "'Please don't call me and please don't say something personal to me because I am so vulnerable you are making it worse.' . . . I mean the one thing I couldn't take was the puppy dog look."

We did come up with a few techniques to reinforce our resolve and our ability to keep our emotional control intact at work. We set up "signals" for coworkers. It was our way of controlling both input from those around us, and our response. A couple of us had a spouse or colleague "run interference" for us by screening well-wishers. Some of us firmly set limits on the number of lunches and meetings requested by sympathetic coworkers and friends. We all used humor and nonsensical analogies to divert intense, sober encounters with well-meaning colleagues and friends. We told people directly that their sympathy was really making things worse. We put the word out that we would appreciate cards—so we would not have to look someone in the eye and start crying. And, more than anything else, we cried at home.

6

Sex and Intimacy

"A lot of the difficult times, like the mutilation of the surgery, the hair loss, feeling so unattractive and not at all sexy, might have been easier if I'd been alone."
—*Daria Davidson*

A few of us were in relationships at the time of our diagnosis and treatment—some new, others long-standing. Those of us who were in relationships found that we had to articulate the roles we wanted our significant others to play in our breast cancer experience.

Letting our partners know what we expected and needed was very difficult. Some of us have insisted on independence; others find that our significant others adjust well within the parameters we've established.

We made our needs clear and then negotiated those things our partners could or could not do for us. We each had a different set of needs and desires that resulted from our individual experiences with this disease. Some of us wanted our partners to participate fully. Others, accustomed to being in complete control, struggled for self-sufficiency and were troubled by our partner's need to take care of us. We all discovered that it requires courage to tell a person you love to leave you alone in a time of

In a study of over twenty-five thousand cancer patients, researchers determined that marital status has an impact on overall survival. The study was designed to assess the relationships among marital status and diagnosis, treatment, and survival. Investigators demonstrated that being married had a positive effect on overall survival, i.e., married cancer patients have a five-year survival rate that is comparable to nonmarried patients ten years younger.

The higher overall survival rate has at least three contributing factors: married people with cancer tend to be diagnosed at an earlier stage; they receive more definitive or potentially curative therapies; and they demonstrate better overall survival rates, even after controlling for treatment and stage of disease.

Improved survival for married breast cancer patients may be the result of a number of factors including better health habits, shorter delay in seeking medical care, less alcoholism, and less mental illness than in the unmarried population. However, researchers theorize that the most important factors may be the degree of social support available within the marriage framework and the improved socioeconomic status associated with marriage.

Goodwin, J., Hunt, W. C., Key, C. R., et al. "The Effect of Marital Status on Stage, Treatment, and Survival of Cancer Patients." *Journal of the American Medical Association.* 258(21) (1987):3125–30.

crisis. For Daria, that meant asking her husband "not to come with me to the doctor's office for the initial consultation because I really needed to conduct it as another routine matter in my very busy life until I knew that this was no longer routine. However, Chuck did come with me to the hospital the day I had my biopsy, and [the doctor] told us that day that it was malignant. My husband's been completely involved from then on out."

Though we are heterosexual, we recognize and understand that breast cancer can affect lesbian relationships in the same way it can heterosexual relationships. We talked with a number of lesbian women and their partners to more clearly identify the special problems they face in their relationships. Probably the most disturbing aspect of breast cancer for a lesbian and her partner is the fear for both that the partner may also develop breast cancer. There are other major concerns facing lesbian women with cancer, including health-care professionals who refuse to recognize a lesbian partner in the same way they would a heterosexual partner; family members who exclude a partner from active participation during the various stages of the disease and treatment process; and an insurance industry that generally does not recognize a lesbian partner as a dependent, which may make the financial burdens even greater for lesbian couples than for heterosexual couples. Most other problems were, however, very similar regardless of sexual preference.

Defining the Roles

It is sometimes easier to give in to a partner's needs, to allow that person to assume the role of nurturer and protector. But some of us found that position to be alien and uncomfortable. We have been trained to focus on problems and to solve them—the more important the problem, the greater the effort. Diversions and distractions are not appreciated. And if the problem is especially important, delegating primary responsibility for it is out of the question.

A caring partner can sometimes become a "needy" partner—one who distracts us and keeps us from addressing the issues. For some of us, the last thing we wanted was to meet that person's need to take care of us. Daria's husband "would have been so happy if I'd permitted him to take care of me." But she admits that she is a very controlling person and never leans on anyone. "He wanted to wait on me hand and foot, but I didn't want to be in the patient role. So a lot of my job was to acknowledge his care and also to say, 'It's not okay for you to do that now.' For me, the control issue was always there."

Joy also feels the need to remain in control. When she was in the hospital for nine days for her first mastectomy, her husband took off work and literally stayed by her side. "It became too much for me." She says she loved him dearly but wasn't willing to turn over control to him. If it hadn't been for a friend who understood her need for personal space, she doesn't think she would have survived it. Her friend said, "Joy, I'll get him out of here!"

Sometimes our zealous partners managed to irritate us even beyond our admittedly strained tolerance levels. Daria's husband kept saying "*we*—'We've got to get through chemo,' and 'We've got to get through the weekend,' and 'We're throwing up every minute.'" She finally told him, "'Wait a second, Chuck. This is not a "we" thing. This is me.' It annoyed me that he was claiming ownership of my experience. He felt that he was going through all of this, too. He was going through something, but it wasn't the same thing I was going through. I told him, 'I'm the one in the boxing ring. You're standing on the sidelines giving me support. And I appreciate that support, don't get me wrong, but it's not the same thing. This is my fight.'"

Others of us had a different story to tell—one of mind-melding support from our partners, an enhancement of strength rather than a drain. Donna's story highlighted for us the uniqueness of each of our approaches to the experience—the accommodations and the limits we have typically associated with our dealings with our partners. She welcomed her husband's full participation. "My husband and I have always leaned on each other so much that it's hard sometimes to differentiate between the two of us in times of crisis. I've never had to struggle with him in terms of how much he would or would not do for me. He has acted as my caretaker, for example, waking me up every few hours during chemotherapy to take my medications. When I was drained and bald and felt like I looked so awful, how wonderful it was to be able to lean on Mark and trust him to protect me when I was vulnerable."

In contrast to some others of our group, Donna appreciated her husband's very personal identification with her disease. She overheard him say to someone that "we just finished chemotherapy," and she thought it was wonderful that he felt so involved. "I could have managed breast cancer without him. I could do it from now on without him, if I had to. Yet I feel exceptionally fortunate to have someone who is there, who doesn't take away my independence, who doesn't rob me of anything. I think the deepening of our relationship is part of the growth process I've experienced with breast cancer."

Though Sally did not live with her significant other, she found that he was invaluable during her experience with her stem-cell transplant. A stem-cell transplant is a significant step in the treatment process, and Sally was particularly afraid of going through it alone. Her friend, Jim, was with her "one hundred percent." When the issue of a

The emphasis on the psychosocial effects of breast cancer has led to a redefinition of the parameters of the disease. Breast cancer studies have demonstrated that for married women, breast cancer is a disease that impacts both members of the couple.

A study designed to assess the long-term adjustment of fourteen couples to breast cancer demonstrated that these marriages were characterized by extraordinarily high levels of enmeshment. They were extremely close emotionally, were closely tied psychologically, and shared an openness of experience that indicated a lack of personal boundaries. Researchers found these couples to be less rigid in their definitions of roles, they had clear and empathetic communication, and demonstrated good listening skills. The findings indicated that no apparent psychological damage occurs over time to the husband or the breast cancer survivor. However, the marriage system does show effects such as loss of personal autonomy as a result of the high degree of cohesion. Such a high degree of cohesion is generally characteristic of marriages having serious problems such as alcoholism or mental illness.

The researchers theorize that because both spouses, individually, were free from psychological disturbances, that extremes of cohesion within the marriage framework may be a method of adapting to the threat of breast cancer.

Carter, R. E., Carter, C. A., Siliunas, M. "Marital Adaptation and Interaction of Couples after a Mastectomy." *Journal of Psychosocial Oncology.* 11(2) (1993):69–81.

transplant first came up, she asked him if he would go with her to her physician's office to talk about it. She believed a transplant would interfere with his life almost as much as it would hers. She was surprised that he readily agreed to go with her; he came with a whole list of questions and talked more than she did. "From that day on, he was so involved in the whole process I was overwhelmed. His involvement has amazed me and impressed me so much I want to cry every time I think about it. He was there helping me get checked into the hospital. He drove to Miami every night after work to be with me, even though I was groggy and full of medicine. He was willing to contact people he didn't even know to give them an update on my condition. He was willing to do anything and everything."

Amy met her new husband in 1986. As she relates, "During the time I was leaving the Wall Street firm and setting up my own business, I met a man through a mutual friend. I smile when I remember that I told him about my breast cancer (which was still new to me) on our second date. He took it calmly and in stride, having had a bad scare himself (that turned out okay), but it shook him to his boots in a way familiar to disaster survivors. He was understanding, smart, funny, warm, and incredibly handsome. We were married in 1990."

New Relationships

Different issues arose for those of us who were in new relationships when our breast cancer was diagnosed. We found that we were discriminating in the things we were willing to share with our partners. It seems there were at least two dimensions to our approaches: We were either greedy about our privacy and hesitant about opening ourselves to degrees of intimacy for which we were not prepared; or we felt a need to protect our partners from having to commit to and become involved with something they themselves could not handle.

Evaluating new relationships:

- assess which current relationships best meet your needs under your current circumstances
- evaluate new relationships to ensure they meet your current needs
- ask your new partner at what level of involvement he or she is comfortable
- share your needs and expectations with your partner
- be flexible—your needs may change

Experiencing breast cancer forced us to take a closer look at this "new" person, to evaluate to what extent we wanted him involved, and then to talk candidly with him about it. Carol S. had a new man in her life whom she'd known for only five months. He immediately became involved in gathering information and going to doctors' appointments with her. She said that though he was caring and wonderful, "during chemotherapy I didn't want him to hang out with me in the bathroom." She felt it might destroy a new relationship, and he respected her feelings. "We worked it out that my friends went with me for my treatments and he didn't visit me that day or the next day. I wanted that separation in a new relationship."

A diagnosis of breast cancer made us acutely aware of the value of time, and some of us chose not to spend our time in a relationship that did not meet our needs.

Cathy's second episode of breast cancer had a negative effect on a relatively new (six-month) relationship. She realized before the mastectomy that there were barriers to communication between them. "He was a very quiet person, not a talker, and we weren't always in sync emotionally. He was comfortable and fun to be with, but we had begun to discuss our religious differences when my cancer recurred." When Cathy found herself facing an emotional crisis, she found she was turning more and more toward her closer family and friends, with whom she could talk more openly. It became evident that this was not a relationship she wanted for the long term. "We actually stayed together as friends through my surgeries, and for several months afterward, but the recurrence made me reassess our relationship, perhaps earlier than I would have otherwise. It became quite clear to me that this man wasn't my soul mate. I wasn't disappointed, really . . . just aware that this was how it was."

Old Relationships

Several of us are divorced but remain in touch with our former husbands. When we got our diagnoses, these men gave us support and encouragement, and it was gratifying. Carol W. stays in close contact with her ex-husband. As Carol recounts, "When he found out about my diagnosis, he called and chewed me out long-distance because I hadn't told him. We have a good relationship, and he wants to be aware of what is going on in my life. It is good knowing and feeling that people are there for me if I want them to be."

Former husbands also can act as an important support system for our children. Carol S.'s former husband and her son helped each other deal with her diagnosis. And

Betsy's former husband sent her flowers in the hospital and called periodically thereafter, sharing information. "It was special because it said 'we're still friends and I care about you.' We are both very involved with our daughters, and so it was important to me that he understood and was supportive."

Enduring Relationships

A solid relationship is likely to remain the same or even be strengthened by having to deal with the stress of a life-threatening illness. In general, the viability of our marriages and intimate relationships was not influenced by our diagnosis, and published research tends to underscore our experience. We found that the nature of our relationships with our partners and significant others before our diagnoses determined our relationships afterward. Our personalities and responsibilities remained relatively the same. In some cases, we suspect our partners may have wanted us to relinquish some of our independence so they could take care of us, but we retained our self-sufficiency, our determination, and our drive. If our partners had a strong, commanding presence, that force continued throughout our experience; if they had been flexible and yielding to our needs before the diagnosis, that did not change.

We must, however, emphasize that the intensity of our relationships increased, irrespective of their previous form and function. We all had an infusion of drama into our relationships, and although it could occasionally be distressing, it more often was rewarding and invigorating.

Donna says that her marriage "went from black and white to Technicolor" as she and her husband faced the crisis of breast cancer together. The experience of her stem-cell transplant demonstrated to Sally the deep commitment of her significant other. Before her transplant, she wondered what kind of commitment he felt toward her because "we'd been playmates more than anything else." But she learned that first month just how much commitment he felt and demonstrated even though "he still won't verbalize it."

Communication

Not surprisingly, communication with our partners and significant others became even more important following our diagnoses of breast cancer. Some of us found that communicating effectively became more difficult and complicated and that our level of communication changed. Betsy became particularly careful about how she talked to her new husband about issues surrounding her diagnosis. As Betsy says, "He is very caring and he is trying very hard, but there is an edge now. It's not that we don't communicate well, but he wants everything to be all right, he doesn't want to hear me say, 'I have a headache. Could it be brain cancer?'"

Other issues to consider:

- you may be confused about your feelings, making them difficult to communicate
- you may need a period of time to internally process your feelings—it is okay to delay discussing them until you are ready
- your partner may be unwilling or unable to discuss certain aspects of your illness

Family members' adaptation to a cancer patient's illness may be characterized by a series of tasks relating to powerlessness, ambivalence, advocacy, age-specific conflicts, uncertainty, and role restructuring. Each of these tasks offers challenges for the cancer survivor as well as the people who love her.

- Powerlessness—family members, as well as patients, may feel powerless in the face of a life-threatening illness. Contrary to expectation, the longer the disease is present, the more powerless they may feel.
- Ambivalence—reaction to long-term illness may include ambivalent feelings towards the patient. These feelings tend to emerge after the crisis of diagnosis or surgery. Ambivalence is generally not a permanent feeling but may require professional assistance to resolve.
- Advocacy—loved ones must advocate for the needs of the patient as well as their own needs, which may be neglected.
- Uncertainty—is a daily part of living with cancer. The possibility of recurrence is always present.
- Age-specific conflicts—cancer patients and their families have more than one life. They face the life of the cancer patient and all of its associated tasks, as well as the normal developmental tasks of a family.
- Role-restructuring—families of cancer patients often find themselves taking on new roles and areas of responsibility. This can be especially difficult for younger family members.

Lewis, F. M. "Family Needs with Long-term Cancer Survivors: What Do We Know, Where Do We Go?" *Proceedings of the American Cancer Society Fourth National Conference on Human Values and Cancer.* New York, New York. (1984): 108–17.

- a third party, e.g., your doctor, counselor, or clergy, may be beneficial in helping you and your partner communicate about uncomfortable issues

There have been issues that we were unwilling to talk about until we had done some additional "processing." We needed to be able to pick the time to discuss issues we considered particularly sensitive, which meant some of our partners had to wait until we were ready to talk. We suspect that some of them didn't mind waiting, that they may have been afraid that if they "opened the door, all of these demons—all our fears and worries—would jump out."

Communication was sometimes a problem for our partners as well. Joy's husband had always found it diffi-cult to communicate verbally, and her cancer exacerbated this trait. "He knew the doctor had said I was terminal, but he was in total denial. He told me that I wasn't to say one more word about cancer, about fear, about dying. He said, 'You're not going to die. You're going to outlive me.'"

Special Issues
for Those Who Are Single

Relationships for unmarried couples involve some issues that need special attention. It was important to us that our significant others be allowed to participate, without hindrance, in our treatment and care decisions, so we dis-cussed this with our family members. We executed legal documents to circumvent difficulties.

Sally addressed many of these issues before she checked into the hospital for her stem-cell transplant. She talked first to hospital administrators to make sure the hospital would accept Jim as if he were a family member. She then spoke with her brother to ensure that Jim was included in any decision making related to her care. She wrote both a standard will and a living will, and gave copies to Jim and to her brother. And she explained to her doctor that Jim was her significant other and she wanted him to be involved in every aspect of her treatment and care.

Sexuality

Whether we agree or not, breasts—subtly or overtly—are identified with sexuality in our society. How we deal with this fact depends on our individual beliefs. Our sexuality may be influenced by treatments that sap our strength, deflate our spirits, and cause physical changes that may affect our libido. For some of us, these changes and challenges cause difficulties, while for others they intensify and complement the physical bond.

It is important to:

- recognize the significance of your breasts to your sexuality and self-image
- acknowledge the physical side effects from treatment, including loss of libido
- understand the sexual dynamic of your relationships
- discuss sexual issues with your partner
- report physical side effects to your health-care team

Breasts, Sexuality, and Self-Image

Dealing with the changes in our physical appearance as the result of lumpectomy or mastectomy seemed to be the least significant sexual issue for us. Cathy still wore the same bathing suit she wore before her mastectomy, and she looks better than before because she has taken better care of the rest of her body. Joy is not concerned about body image because of her mastectomies. "My breasts aren't who I am. I'm not afraid of someone seeing my body." Carol H. adds that she "chose not to have reconstruction after the partial mastectomy. I was really hung up on the scars after the radical groin dissection, but this time I just said it was okay to be me the way I was."

Whether we were involved with a sexual partner at the time of our diagnosis or not, the concerns some of us felt about being in a sexual relationship seemed to center around issues other than body image. One of these issues was that a sexual relationship seemed "irrelevant" in our lives. We didn't yearn for this type of companionship. Another was the difficulty we had in getting past the fear of recurrence and of doing "damage" that could bring about a relapse. And Betsy recalls, "My husband wanted to see my lumpectomy scar as soon as it was feasible, and he had no problems. I was the one who had problems. I didn't like touching my breast or having anyone else touch it. I protected and guarded it. I didn't want a bruise or anything that would cause another cancer. That attitude has slowly changed."

Cathy says, "Because of my Christian beliefs, I have been celibate for many years. When I found out I was going to lose my breast, my boyfriend and I were not involved sexually. Even though it goes against my religious beliefs, I have to admit that I did give some thought to whether or not I wanted to 'do it' while I still had both of my natural breasts. I knew sex probably wouldn't be the same for me after surgery, but I decided to stick with my faith, and I don't regret it. Celibacy is difficult, and keeps people at a distance, but it keeps me in emotional control, which is how I feel most comfortable."

Physical Changes

The physical side effects of treatment affected our desire for and satisfaction from sexual experiences more than did the changes in our physical appearance. Some of the physical side effects we experienced as a result of breast cancer therapy included a lack of feeling in the treated breast, vaginal dryness, premature menopause, a decrease in libido, and a lack of vaginal sensitivity during intercourse. Chemotherapy seemed to create the most negative consequences for us.

Possible physical changes, many of which are temporary, include:

- loss of feeling in the treated breast
- vaginal dryness
- premature menopause
- lack of vaginal sensitivity during intercourse
- decreased libido

Some of us have experienced a decrease in libido following chemotherapy, which is not unusual, as chemotherapy causes a decrease in androgen levels, and androgens drive the libido. Betsy relates, "One of my real regrets is that I just don't have the same level of sexual

Historically, breast cancer has been thought of as traumatic to a woman's sexual functioning, including aspects such as feelings of attractiveness, femininity, and desire. Mastectomies were thought to be frequent precursors to divorce or relationship termination. Breast-conserving treatment and breast reconstruction were thought to have a significant impact on the reduction of these feelings.

Recently, however, studies have indicated that the major sexual dysfunction affecting breast cancer survivors is not the removal of the breast, but premature menopause and its associated symptoms.

For many premenopausal women diagnosed with breast cancer each year, chemotherapy and/or antiestrogenic therapies can bring about irreversible premature menopause. Symptoms associated with premature menopause include loss of vaginal lubrication, hot flashes, and eventual atrophy of the vagina.

In addition, women undergoing chemotherapy must cope with the physical changes that it brings, such as hair loss, weight gain, and nausea.

Schover, L. "The Impact of Breast Cancer on Sexuality, Body Image, and Intimate Relationships." *CA—A Cancer Journal for Clinicians.* 41(2) (1991):112–20.

desire. I've always been a sexy person. If I was walking down the street and saw a guy with great legs, I'd think about what it would be like to sleep with him. Now that impulse is gone. I had the chemo and the radiation, and after a while, I stopped feeling tired and got back to normal life, but my sexual desire didn't come back. Is it because I'm in premature menopause or because I'm still worried about cancer and can't relax? Maybe it's a combination. It is hard to think about sex when you are worried about dying. It is just not a priority."

> A decrease in libido may be the result of treatment, stress, fatigue, anxiety, and/or medications. Each of these factors needs careful evaluation, by the breast cancer patient, her partner, and her medical team, to facilitate an improvement in sexual function.
>
> Auchincloss, S. S. "Sexual Dysfunction in Cancer Patients: Issues in Evaluation and Treatment." *Handbook of Psychooncology*. Eds. Holland, J. C., Rowland, J. H. Oxford University Press. New York, New York. 1990.

In addition to a decrease in sexual desire, some of us experienced a loss of vaginal sensitivity during intercourse. As Daria told her husband, "Guys don't like to wear condoms because they lose sensitivity. Think about having sex with a Goodyear tire on your penis. That's how much sensitivity I've lost."

We want to emphasize that not all of us have experienced negative effects on our sex lives as a result of the disease and treatment. Sexuality continues to be a special, vital, and integral part of our lives. We all feel the need for intimacy, affection, social interaction, and touch.

Talking About It

Those of us who are involved in intimate relationships involving sexual interaction found that more communication was required to let our partners know how we felt following our treatment for breast cancer. Carol S. had difficulty, first with breast tenderness, then with her own unwillingness to be touched. She noted that "communicating these subtle things to your lover isn't easy."

Daria acknowledges that, even now, sex is sometimes a problem for her, even though she and her husband have a very open relationship and communicate well. Her husband tries to please her, but she is just not as sensitive as she used to be. "I finally had to tell him, 'It's not going to happen for me. And the more you try, the worse it makes me feel, so just go with it. I'm okay.' But it's not okay for him because he'd like sex to be great for both of us."

The Sexual Dynamic

We have considered whether it is better to be in an intimate sexual relationship during the diagnosis and treatment for breast cancer or whether it is better to be alone. Our feelings about this are complex and include anxiety about how our decisions will affect our partners, concern about whether and how much we should worry about our partners' feelings, and the stress of just having to deal with these troublesome issues. Cathy relates that "the first time I had breast cancer, I didn't have a significant other, so I didn't have to be concerned about what the possibility of losing my breast would mean to him. I was really grateful that I didn't have to worry about that. I could focus solely on my own feelings." Carol S. was "worried about making the decision of a lumpectomy versus a mastectomy around the man in my life. It bothered me as a feminist. There were times when I wished I didn't have someone in my life so I could feel absolutely clear that it was my own decision." For Betsy, "When the choice had to be made about a mastectomy or a lumpectomy, my husband gave me permission to do what I wanted. There was no pressure from him. But his image of me was very important. He is definitely a 'tits' man! I don't know if that influenced my decision."

While appreciating the support she received from her husband, Daria wondered if it might have been easier to

Breast cancer and all the changes it brings about can affect every area of a woman's life, including sexuality. The following are some tips for regaining sexual confidence after cancer:

- emphasize the positive aspects of your physical and emotional self
- choose an appropriate time for sexual togetherness; try to be rested and free from distractions
- wear comfortable yet attractive clothing; make yourself feel good about your appearance
- try a warm shower together
- set the mood with wine, candles, and music
- body massage can be stimulating to both partners
- find a position that is comfortable and will not be tiring
- use a lubricant, if needed
- if necessary, use a prescribed pain medication or muscle relaxant to make sexual activity more comfortable
- conserve energy for sex; delegate some household chores to others
- communicate with your partner
- consider a support group or a counselor if problems do not ease with time
- take time and initiative to explore the many ways to express physical love and desire

Grier, S. "Sexuality and Women with Cancer: Nursing Implications." *Oncology Patient Care.* 3(1) (1992):5–9.

go through treatment without considering relationship issues. "I am in a relationship and I am committed to the relationship, and my husband is incredibly supportive. But sometimes I wonder if the whole experience of treatment might have been easier if I'd been alone. A lot of the difficult times, like the mutilation of the surgery, the hair loss, feeling so unattractive and not at all sexy, might have been easier if I'd been alone. I could have ignored the sexuality issues if it had just been me. I could have gone about my business with the chemo and not have tried to be a sexual person, too. I could have focused on just getting through it."

7

The Genetic Strand—
The Tie That Binds

*"If one of my daughters develops breast cancer fifteen
or twenty years from now, and I have to go through all
this again, and there are still no answers, look out!"*
—*Betsy Lambert*

The anguish of breast cancer is not limited to the women
it strikes. Rather, generations of families are caught in a
web of fear, guilt, and anxiety caused by the disease. Our
grandmothers and mothers worry that they may be partly
responsible for our diagnoses, perhaps by transmitting a
genetic predisposition to the disease. In turn, we worry
that we have created a dreadful legacy that will affect our
daughters and granddaughters. As Amy says, "Breast
cancer advocates are concerned about the legacy of breast
cancer, and we are working to change the state of knowledge and find the cause and the cure for this disease to
protect our daughters." Our sisters worry that they will
be next. Recent studies suggest that the genetic link is not
limited just to the female side of the family—fathers also
can carry and transmit the responsible gene, and mothers
can pass the gene to sons as well as daughters.

Our parents are terrified that they will lose us; after all, we are supposed to outlive them. Our children also fear that they will lose us. Our daughters, in particular, are fearful that one day they will be diagnosed with breast cancer. Yet though our illness deeply affects the well-being of those we love, we can only watch.

Our Parents

The risk of developing breast cancer is higher for women who have a family history of cancer, particularly for women whose mothers or sisters have had breast cancer. Our individual risk profiles for developing breast cancer ranged from having no family history of cancer, to having a father who died from prostate cancer, to having lost mothers and grandmothers to breast cancer. Of the ten women in our group, five were the first in their extended family to develop breast cancer. Joy had two first cousins who were diagnosed with breast cancer shortly after her diagnosis; they both died relatively quickly. Sometimes breast cancer skips a generation. Cathy's mother has not

---

Numerous studies have demonstrated a two-fold increase in risk for women with a mother or sister diagnosed with breast cancer. For a woman with both a mother and sister with breast cancer the risk is fourteen times that of a woman with no familial breast disease.

Wellisch, D. K., Gritz, E. R., Schain, W., et al. "Psychological Functioning of Daughters of Breast Cancer Patients." Part 1: Daughters and comparison subjects. *Psychosomatics.* 32(3) (1991):324–36.

developed breast cancer, but her grandmother died from the disease.

Genetic risks:

- a family history of cancer increases a woman's risk of developing breast cancer
- a history of breast cancer in a mother or sister significantly increases a woman's risk of developing breast cancer; on the other hand, 80 percent of breast cancer patients have no family history of breast cancer
- women whose fathers have prostate cancer have a fourfold risk of developing breast cancer

Both Daria's and Sally's mothers were diagnosed with breast cancer when they were in their sixties, and both died of the disease. Daria's mother was diagnosed at age sixty-two with the same kind of tumor as Daria's. Her mother had two positive lymph nodes compared to Daria's single node involvement, and she was treated with the standard six months of chemotherapy with CMF. Ten months later, the cancer had metastasized to her lung and bone, and she died soon after. Her grandmother also had breast cancer. Naturally, when Daria began to compare her statistics to that of her mother she feared she "would be dead by Christmas."

By the time Sally's mother was diagnosed at age sixty-eight, her breast cancer had metastasized and was inoperable. She died three years after the diagnosis, and Sally cared for her the last several months. She says, "Mother's experience made me realize that I was at risk and had to be vigilant, but I had no idea that breast cancer would strike me so soon. Because of my vigilance, I thought I'd been fortunate enough to catch the cancer in time. But I hadn't. My experience with her cancer taught me so much and helped prepare me for my own cancer. Mom's living her cancer with graciousness and courage served as a wonderful role model."

Telling our mothers about our diagnosis and anticipating their responses was a source of major concern and anxiety for all of us. We tried to think of ways to make it easier for them and for ourselves. Carol H. describes her experiences: "My mom lives in Florida, I in New Jersey, so my breast cancer news was shared over the phone. My mother had just lost her third child, there were three of us left . . . a healthy younger brother, a younger brother who had thyroid cancer, and me. She had cared for me when I had my melanoma surgeries. . . . I cried as I shared with Mom, part for me, and for her and all of the sadness she had experienced in her time." Some of us carefully planned how we would tell our mothers about our diagnoses in order to minimize their distress and protect ourselves from their emotions. Carol S. scripted the conversation she planned to have with her mother. Her son suggested that he fly to her mother's house in Los Angeles so that he could offer her mother emotional support and help her deal with the news when Carol called to tell her about her cancer for the first time. At that point, her sister, Barbara, and her family, who live near Carol's mother, were ready to step in after Carol's son returned to England. This was a unique approach to communicating the diagnosis to an elderly mother.

Telling your mother about your diagnosis:

- will warrant careful planning
- may make it important to find ways to protect yourself from her emotional response
- may cause her to feel partly responsible for your disease if you have a family history of cancer

- means it may be particularly difficult for her to think you may die before she does
- may cause her to manifest feelings of guilt, fear, and overwhelming sadness
- will probably intensify your relationship with her, whether positive or negative, after diagnosis and during treatment
- will require you to be prepared to deal with her need to help and to take care of you
- will require you to concentrate on what makes you strong and avoid those emotions that sap your strength

The news of our diagnoses was even more difficult for those of our mothers who believed that their genes were partly responsible for our disease. It was particularly hard for Cathy's mother because she believed that Cathy's cancer was somehow her fault. Even though she herself does not have breast cancer, her mother did, and the gene was passed on to Cathy.

While Betsy has no history of cancer on her mother's side of the family, her father was diagnosed with prostate cancer that metastasized to other parts of his body. He died shortly after diagnosis. It surprised Betsy to learn that any history of cancer in the family increases a person's risk, and that women whose fathers have had prostate cancer are four times as likely to have breast cancer. And even though the connection was on the paternal side, her mother still responded with guilt. "It's all my fault. I should never have married your father!"

In addition to feeling guilty for the genes they have given us, some of our mothers said they wished they had been diagnosed with breast cancer instead of us. Like most mothers, they would gladly be ill themselves rather than have to watch their children suffer. It is difficult to think about losing a child, and many mothers say, "If only it could be me."

Our mothers fear they will lose us. We've all heard women say that it's not right that a mother should have to watch her child die—and we believe it. Many of us have thought the same thing about our own children! Nevertheless, our mothers' fears of our deaths is a difficult issue for us and one that cannot be easily resolved. Betsy explains, "My mother can't bear to think that she might lose her only daughter. It scares her to think that she may outlive me. We can't talk about it, except on a very limited basis, because it's such an explosive issue. The problem is, there is no solution; there is no way we will know the answer until one of us dies."

Guilt, fear, and overwhelming sadness were the predominant themes in our mothers' responses to our illness. Those feelings were just the beginning; they were acted out in a variety of ways that occasionally made our days easier but more often made them trying. There is something especially poignant about the mother-daughter connection, whether the mother is still living or not and whether the relationship is positive and strong or strained and annoying.

Cathy's primary concern with her first diagnosis, and on recurrence, was her mother and how she would take the news. The bond between the two of them is very strong, and Cathy was willing to take on her mother's concerns and emotions—their relationship had always been mutually supportive. "Giving" to her mother at this time was a source of strength to Cathy. Her mother suggested going to a healing service conducted by one of the nationally known Christian healing ministers she watched on television. Cathy realized that her mother needed to feel that she could help in some way, so she went with her mother to Louisiana to attend a healing service. "The trip to Baton Rouge was meaningful to both of us. To Mom, it meant that we'd done everything within our power to ensure my future health. It was important to me, as a Christian, to have others lay hands on me and pray for my healing. It was a special time for Mom and me to be together, away from all the doctors, to focus on 'healing of the soul,' not only the body. I felt good about going because it made my mom feel there was something she could do to help me. And it did help. After that trip, I felt at peace and certain that I was doing the right thing."

For some of us, our concern for our mothers' emotional state surpassed even our concern for ourselves. But for others, our illness intensified some uncomfortable issues. In general, we believe that our interactions with our mothers after our diagnosis followed the pattern of our relationship prior to breast cancer. Those of us who had troublesome relationships with our mothers before our diagnosis found that things remained much the same following diagnosis. As one of us relates, "Long before I had breast cancer, there were certain things my mom and I couldn't talk about . . . we've just had to stay away from certain topics because we disagree so much. That makes dealing with the issues surrounding my breast cancer all the more difficult." Another says, "My relationship with my mother has been tough all my life. We're just too different. It's not that I don't love her, but I don't want her involved in my daily life. Since my diagnosis, it has become difficult because she wants to mother me, and that makes me angry. I know that some people respond to a life-threatening situation by making attempts to fix relationships. But I have no motivation whatsoever to do that. I don't want to spend my energy trying to satisfy my mother's emotional needs. I want her to seek support from others in the family instead of draining me dry."

For those of us in difficult mother-daughter relationships, the prospect of having "my mother come and take care of me was the last thing in the world I wanted or needed." Managing our mothers' emotions made some of us feel drained and angry. One of us says, "I wasn't going to tell my mother about my diagnosis at all because I felt that her emotions would be so exhausting. I thought the best way to take care of myself was not to tell her. Not to worry her. I knew that her first response would be to fly to my home and take care of me, and having her here would require so much energy on my part."

Some of us may sound cold and unfeeling when we talk about how trying some of our mothers became to us during this time. But it is important to understand that we did recognize their distress, and that they wanted and needed to be able to do something to help us. At the risk of excusing our attitudes, we emphasize that we were not and are not cavalier in our relationships with our mothers, but this became a time for us to confront our own feelings—in some cases for the first time—about our mothers. If there is a theme that predominates here, it is that we strongly believe that it is important to concentrate on ourselves now and to look to those things that bolster our strength rather than weaken us.

Those of us who financially support our parents have an additional worry. What will happen to them if we die before they do? As planners and problem solvers, we want to make arrangements now to ensure that our parents are secure. But arranging for their futures isn't easy. After all, it is not particularly pleasant to have to change a lifestyle to accommodate a daughter's concerns about her own illness. As her mother's main economic resource, Carol S. wants to be sure her mother is taken care of if something happens to her. She wishes, especially when she is feeling down, that her mother would make the decision to move to a nursing home that offers graduated care but takes only people when they are well. But at eighty-four her mother is active, healthy, loves her independence, and does not want to change her life.

Pregnancy Following Treatment for Breast Cancer

The question of whether to become pregnant after being diagnosed and treated for breast cancer is still a major concern. Amy relates, "Family was important for both of us, maybe because we were both only children. We periodically discussed having children, and of course, I was concerned about what my breast cancer diagnosis meant in terms of bearing children." Amy's position at NABCO, which she assumed in 1990, allowed her access to most of the available information on breast cancer research, but because of the frustrating state of that research, there were no clear answers available. Amy went to friends in the oncology community and her own medical team for guidance. She learned that, in their collective opinion, pregnancy was not necessarily a high-risk proposition for a woman with early-stage breast cancer who had passed the two- to three-year window after surgery (when recurrence is most likely). This theory has since been confirmed by the National Cancer Institute in a retrospective study. Pregnancy under these conditions is, however, not

Until recently, pregnancy after mastectomy was thought to have an adverse effect on survival for breast cancer patients. Recent studies, however, have found that pregnancy after treatment for breast cancer has no demonstrable negative effect on prognosis. This study of 578 breast cancer patients demonstrated a slight improvement in survival for those women becoming pregnant after mastectomy. With more women delaying childbirth and being diagnosed with breast cancer at earlier ages, childbirth after treatment for breast cancer is an area ripe for further study.

Ariel, I. M., Kempner, R. "The Prognosis of Patients Who Become Pregnant After Mastectomy for Breast Cancer." *International Surgery.* 74 (1989):185–87.

completely without risk. After long deliberation and soul-searching, Amy decided to try to get pregnant. Her son, Henry, was born in 1992.

Our Children

We all have close and loving relationships with our children. Six of us were single parents for at least a portion of our children's lives, and this made us even closer to our children. Amy is the newest mother. As she recalls, "Every mother thinks her son is the most wonderful, astonishing, perfect being. Somehow, being a mother who has survived breast cancer makes my baby even more of a miracle. He is the essence of life: the smell of his hair, the way he laughs when I tickle him, the way he greets me with a big "Hi!" at night, as if I am the center of his world. I wonder if I would appreciate him so intensely if I didn't have the past that I do. Of course, I'll never know."

For the rest of us with children, the diagnosis of breast cancer occurred when they were teenagers or older, although Carol H. had a previous cancer diagnosis—malignant melanoma, which she continues to battle today—when her sons were in elementary school. For the three of us who have children and who were in relationships with significant others at the time of our diagnosis, our relationships with our children took on an even greater significance. Our diagnosis made us concerned about them, especially about their fear of losing us and their fear of their own risk of getting cancer. We have no choice but to watch as this burden of worry and fear, a burden imposed by our illness, forces our sons and daughters to face the realities of life sooner than they otherwise would have. This created in some of us nagging feelings of guilt. We felt guilty about disrupting our children's lives, about causing them emotional distress and pain, and particularly, if our immediate family did not have a history of cancer, about starting a new legacy that might afflict our children and their children. Carol W. explains, "There was no cancer on either my mother's or father's side of the family as far as I know. I feel like I started a tradition—a terrible tradition that I hope ends with me."

Thoughts on the genetic link:

- don't be surprised if you feel guilty about what your diagnosis means to your children, but try to let go of the guilt—this is not something you can control
- you will probably be able to predict your children's reactions, which will include fear, anxiety, pragmatism, encouragement, avoidance

- you may need to tailor your talks with your children to enable each one to exhibit his/her strengths and thus support you in ways most helpful to you
- your children will be afraid of losing you
- your daughters may be particularly afraid of their own risk for developing breast cancer
- prophylactic mastectomy for young women at high risk is controversial, but it is often considered as an option to women with high familial risk

Joy recalls that on the day of her initial diagnosis, "The worst part was thinking about my two daughters. I kept thinking about how I had breast cancer and I'd given them my genes and did that mean I'd also given them breast cancer?"

One of the most difficult aspects of learning about our diagnosis was knowing what it implied in terms of our daughters' risk for the disease. Daria is the mother of identical twins, who "are extremely worried about developing breast cancer. After all, three generations of women in our family have had breast cancer. My daughters said to me, 'We'll just have to get our breasts cut off.' They're only twenty-two!"

One of Betsy's daughters has considered having a prophylactic mastectomy. Carol W.'s daughter, both of Betsy's daughters, and Joy's daughters consulted with their mothers' physicians about their own risk of developing breast cancer and what they can do to minimize that risk, or at least detect the disease as early as possible.

In addition to the fear that they might develop breast cancer one day, our daughters have to cope with the fear of losing us—as do our sons. While each of our children reacted in his or her own unique way to the news of our

Prophylactic mastectomy for patients considered to be at high risk of developing breast cancer remains controversial. For patients considering the procedure, the risk-to-benefit ratio must be carefully considered. The assumption that prophylactic mastectomy eliminates all further risk of breast cancer is unfounded.

In most cases of prophylactic mastectomy, a subcutaneous mastectomy is performed. This procedure leaves behind a substantial amount of glandular tissue, which may develop cancerous cells. Although the subcutaneous mastectomy is cosmetically preferred, most surgeons believe that a total mastectomy is superior, if all the glandular elements of the breast can be removed.

In a study done to determine the efficacy of total mastectomy in removing all glandular breast tissue, five high-risk patients were selected. All received a bilateral total mastectomy. In most cases, breast tissue was found to remain after the surgery. The researchers noted that a total glandular extupation is possible with some changes. Mastectomy should be extended to include a layer of pectorals major fascia and into the lower-level axilla. This will ensure the removal of most of the breast tissue.

This operation may be, in principle, a superior method of preventing breast cancer, but patients should continue routine surveillance.

Temple, W. T., Lindsay, R. L., Magi, E., et al. "Technical Consideration for Prophylactic Mastectomy." *American Journal of Surgery.* 161 (1991):413–15.

diagnosis, there seem to be two common patterns. Some of our children were pragmatic and levelheaded, meeting the diagnosis head-on, assuring us that we would be fine. They went with us to visit our physicians and helped us gather information. Carol S.'s son was a source of encouragement, strength, and support for her, and he provided tangible assistance by researching treatment options, helping her with her own mother, and organizing friends to take her to treatment.

Others were too threatened by our diagnosis to deal with it directly. They needed to shield themselves from hearing about our feelings and fears. As one of us relates, "One of my daughters totally lost it. She was terrified that her mother was going to die. My other daughter was very pragmatic. She said, 'Okay, Mom, you are not going to die. I am not going to be without my mother. I know that for sure. It is not in the plan for you to die, so just get your act together.'" Another of us reflects, "One daughter told me that I was going to be okay. She was the problem solver, the nurturer, and less frightened than my other daughter. My other daughter doesn't want to address the idea that she could lose me. She just can't do it. She was too afraid to call and find out the results of my biopsy. She told me later, 'I just couldn't do it. I'm sorry.'"

These differences neither surprised us nor really interfered with our relationships with our children. We appreciate their individual differences, and, although the pragmatic responses were more helpful, it is easy to understand responses of avoidance, fear, and anxiety. Interestingly, we believe that, in general, we were and are less impatient with our children's reactions to our illness than we were with our mothers'!

Most of us get the support and comfort we need from our children. But we find that we have to tailor our talks, depending on their needs. We can say more to one than another. Ultimately, though, they each adjust in their own way.

Returning to our own feelings of guilt, we recognize that one thing this disease insidiously encourages is guilt.

Sixty daughters of women with breast cancer were cross-sectionally studied to determine the effects of their mothers' illness on their psychological functioning. Common emotional themes included: fear of death and/or a mutilated maternal body image; unresolved grief and/or depression; guilt related to time spent with mother; and lowered self-esteem.

Daughters found it difficult to put their mothers' breast cancer behind them, emotionally, thus leading to a perceived change in life course. The impact of the mother's breast cancer can potentially be conceptualized at the interactional level and the representational level.

At the interactional level, breast cancer can invade and change family life. This can incorporate the withdrawal of resources, time, attention, and emotional support from the children. Many times daughters are required to assume the motherly role while the mother is ill. This aspect tends to affect younger children more than older, more self-sufficient children.

At the representational level, the daughter may integrate the image of a sick and potentially dying mother into her own self-image, along with the existing well-mother image. This juxtaposition of images is the basis for the daughter's self-representation in adult life. This can be potentially more serious for adolescent or younger daughters who have not yet solidified their own self-images.

The impact of a mother's breast cancer on daughters encompasses many developmental areas including self-esteem, sexual functioning, and change in roles and life plans.

Wellisch, D. K., Gritz, E. R., Schain, W., et al. "Psychological Functioning of Daughters of Breast Cancer Patients." Part 1: Daughters and comparison subjects. *Psychosomatics*. 32(3) (1991):324–36.

It is too easy for us to take on the responsibility for our parents' and children's feelings or to try to meet their expectations about how we should behave: We should let them help, we should avoid the topic, we should be cheerful, we should be somber, etc., etc., etc. But what better time than now to take a stand? Ultimately, we must try to stop feeling that we are responsible for what happens to our parents and children, or that we can control the events of their lives. Betsy explains, "My daughters' lives will go on. So will my mother's. They will be just fine whether I am here or not. I am pretty clear about that. I don't feel that I need to stay to do things or say things to make their lives work. This is the way it is. This is the way life rolls out. How can I apologize to them? The situation is beyond my control and has been and will continue to be."

You can help your family get through this by:

- letting them share the experience, to the extent that they actually can help you get through it
- trying to be sensitive to the differences in your children, and to honor their preferences for involvement or noninvolvement

However, take care to:

- carefully consider whether you can take on the additional emotional burden of a parent or child who isn't coping particularly well
- remember, you are not responsible for making your family feel okay about your illness
- carefully consider whether you really want your parents or children to organize their lives around taking care of you—even if they insist

- be willing to let your family in, if and when they can help. It is okay to let them be a part of your life.

This also means that we cannot allow our parents or our children to put their own lives on hold for us, no matter how much they would like to do so. We have learned this from experience. As one of us explains, "I allowed my daughter to leave college to take care of me. Eventually I insisted that she move out, go back to school, and get on with her own life. Now I wish I hadn't allowed her to put her life on hold for my sake."

It's not pleasant to think that we may need our children to care for us someday. We do not want to be perceived as weak or vulnerable, and it is difficult for us to admit that we may not be as invincible as we had always assumed. One of the lessons we have tried to learn from our breast cancer experience is to let our guard down and let our children in. Carol W. says, "My daughter is my only child, and we have a close relationship. When I told her about my diagnosis, it was clear to me that she wanted to look out for her mother. I forced myself to allow her to take on that role. I tried not to be my normal controlling self . . . and I had to learn to yield a little bit. Now I keep her apprised of what's going on because, of course, she doesn't allow me not to. So I am learning to allow her to be more a part of what is going on in my life. I am learning to allow her to enter that private space. Perhaps I even owe it to her. After all, she may be the one who has to care for me one day, as I cared for my own mother."

Carol H. and Joy used events in their children's lives as goals during their treatment for cancer. They told themselves, "I just have to make it until . . ." Carol H. used her sons' graduations from high school as goals. And as

A recent discovery of a single gene, BRCA-1, which may be linked to breast cancer, has far-reaching psychological and clinical ramifications. BRCA-1, the breast cancer susceptibility gene, may be carried by one in two hundred women in America today. These women face an 85 percent risk of developing breast cancer, with 50 percent of these cases occurring before the age of fifty. The mutation of the BRCA-1 gene may also be implicated in a higher risk of ovarian cancer in women and prostate cancer in men. The gene is passed down through the generations in the classic Mendelian pattern of autosomal dominant transmission with 50 percent of children of carriers inheriting the BRCA-1 mutation.

Although the majority of cases of breast cancer in women occur without evidence of an inherited increased risk, analyses of tumor specimens suggest that the BRCA-1 gene may also play a role in these cancer cases.

The testing and identification of the BRCA-1 gene has presented new challenges for researchers, genetic counselors, and women with a familial history of breast cancer. Options for women identified as carriers of the gene may include increased surveillance and the more aggressive prophylactic removal of breast and/or ovaries.

This raises questions regarding safeguarding medical records. Concern about the possibility of insurance companies' access to medical records of women carriers of the gene and denying them coverage has caused researchers to keep the records in a private file until a policy is issued.

Biesecker, B. B., Boehnke, M., Calzone, K., et al. "Genetic Counseling for Families with Inherited Susceptibility to Breast and Ovarian Cancer." *Journal of the American Medical Association.* 269(15) (1993):1970–74.

In a recent interview, Dr. Francis Collins discussed some of the implications that the identification of the cancer susceptibility gene, BRCA-1, and others may have in the future. Collins foresees using DNA testing for all patients to assess their risks for genetically linked diseases in the future. Physicians would then be able to give the patients a personalized scheme for preventative medicine.

Dr. Collins is hopeful that, in the future, genetic testing will be useful in a preventive manner, using nontoxic genetic therapies to treat diseases and prevent potentially fatal outcomes. He states, "I believe that our research gains will greatly decrease the possibility of any tragic aspects."

Roberts, L. "Zeroing in on a Breast Cancer Susceptibility Gene." *Science.* 259 (1993):622–25.

Joy explains, "I've had to pick a minigoal, like a grandchild being born, or my daughters getting married. It's always short-term, so it's something that's going to happen in the next six months."

Comments on the Genetic Link

A good deal of current research points to the presence of a gene that may be linked to breast cancer. Because the discovery of the genetic link for risk of breast cancer is so new, only a limited number of facilities are involved in these studies. Women interested in participating in genetic research should discuss their familial history with their oncology team to determine their risk factors and what

As the race to map the human genetic code intensifies, investigators find themselves on the edge of a new horizon in medical practice. With the discovery of the breast cancer susceptibility gene, BRCA-1, a plethora of questions arise. Investigators have already identified which women in a few cancer-prone families carry the gene. Now they are faced with a new set of challenges regarding the disclosure of this information to women carrying the gene and the subsequent counseling and options available to these women.

Geneticists Barbara Welser and Francis Collins at the University of Michigan at Ann Arbor now run one of the first genetic screening and counseling centers in the world. So far they have counseled about fifty members of one breast cancer–prone family. They have assembled a team of twelve professionals divided into counseling groups, each consisting of a geneticist, an oncologist, and a genetic counselor. The team meets with the family members after the screening process. Some of the challenges they face include disclosure issues such as what age is appropriate for genetic disclosure (currently status is given at age eighteen), exactly how solid the data need to be, and concern about insurance companies' use of the information.

Roberts. L. "Genetic Counseling—A Preview of What's in Store." *Science*. 259 (1993):624.

they should do if they are eligible to participate in the studies.

We think that families with a history of breast cancer should know about genetic research. And as the research progresses, blood tests with markers, as well as other procedures that can help a woman manage her genetic risk, may be developed. It is also important to recognize that the genetic link does not explain environmental factors that contribute to risk. Daria and her identical twin daughters went to a medical center in Dallas to have their genetic predisposition for breast cancer assessed. Daria says, "Now the kids know that, just because my mother, my grandmother, and I had breast cancer, does not necessarily mean they are going to get it. So many other risk factors also play a role in developing breast cancer."

8

Dealing with Emotions

"The buzz word is intensity."
—*Donna Cederberg*

The Range of Emotions

From the moment of diagnosis, the experience of breast cancer evokes many emotions: anger, anxiety, depression, sadness, and despair to name a few. We are primarily concerned about how the diagnosis affects our lives to-day—how we manage to fit this new responsibility into a schedule already packed to maximum capacity. We are concerned about how we can maintain the equilibrium we have worked so hard to achieve, knowing that the diagnosis we have been given will create major disruptions in our lives. We also worry about recurrence, death, surgery, and other treatments, and how treatments will affect our self-esteem and self-image. We are disquieted by the possibility of disfigurement. We are apprehensive about maintaining our relationships with our partners and significant others; about being able to care for our children, parents, and others who depend upon us; and about the impact of breast cancer on our careers.

Emotional responses:

- anger
- anxiety
- crying
- despair
- joy

- love
- rage
- rationalization
- sadness
- sense of loss

All of our emotions, from anger and fear to joy and love, seem to be intensified. We wonder how we can carry on at this level of emotional vigor. Donna says, "The buzz word is intensity. I'm tired at night because I feel so much and feel it so intensely. I feel joy and love with the same intensity as fear and rage."

We often find it difficult to allow ourselves to ride the waves of emotions because, as professional women, we're used to putting aside our emotions. We feel more comfortable when we're in our heads—intellectualizing and rationalizing, solving problems, and making decisions. Our culture taught us from an early age to suppress what are considered unpleasant or unacceptable emotions, and our professional environments are generally not conducive to emotional display. Carol H. says, "I wasn't taught what emotions were, much less that I could express them. Anger and other 'not nice' feelings weren't allowed in my family or in the corporate world I grew up in. So I didn't feel my emotions. I said, 'I don't need them.' Even now, I sometimes have to drag out a feeling."

Breast cancer has forced each of us to find ways to deal with our emotions so that we can successfully adjust to our disease and regain control of our lives. We have ad-

Anxiety is such a common reaction to a diagnosis of breast cancer that most health-care professionals regard it as the "normal" reaction during the postdiagnosis phase of treatment. Eighty-five percent of all newly diagnosed patients experience distress during this period. Concerns about death, disfigurement, maintaining family and work responsibilities, and treatment options make this period difficult, at best.

Patients generally react in one of two ways, denial or avoidance. Some studies have suggested that denial of diagnosis may lead to delay in treatment and less acceptance of the situation. Watson, et al. found that denial may be an effective mechanism for reducing the stress associated with the diagnosis of a life-threatening illness. The researchers failed to show a relationship between denial and delay in seeking treatment. They theorize that denial may be a good short-term coping response and that encouraging confrontation and acceptance during the postdiagnosis period does not facilitate better coping.

Watson, M., Greer, S., Blake, S., et al. "Reaction to a Diagnosis of Breast Cancer." *Cancer*. 53 (1984):2008–12.

dressed our emotional needs in a variety of ways, choosing the methods that worked best for us. These methods include individual counseling, support groups, use of imagery and visualization techniques, keeping journals, exercising, expressing and releasing emotions by crying or other physical means, finding positive examples, and looking for support from family and friends. Each of us had to discover the approaches best suited to our own emotional needs at each point in our individual journeys.

We believe it is important to emphasize that although there were similarities in how each of us responded to our diagnosis and then worked through our emotions, there were also differences. These differences can be attributed to our individual life experiences and philosophies. Joy, for example, characterizes herself as "a fighter"—a woman who faces each situation directly and with a determination to win. Donna approaches her disease a little differently, less like a soldier and more like a conscientious objector. She believes that "a fighting spirit" is different from anger, and that fighting has less focus. For Donna, fighting is not always the most effective way to cope with the disease.

Our breast cancer journeys began with the emotional impact of the news of our diagnosis. We believe that hearing the diagnosis was the most devastating moment in our lives. Betsy says she was "totally destroyed." Others of us could find nothing in our lives that came close to the devastation of that moment.

There was an overwhelming feeling of sadness and despair, and, in some cases, that sadness was related to what the diagnosis would mean to our families as well as to us. We found ourselves—and still find ourselves—removed from our own lives, looking down on "this person" who was doing so well, was so successful after having worked so hard, and then saying, "How sad this had to happen to her." It was like watching a very sad movie.

Our despair seemed to originate with what we had heard about cancer, and even those of us with a degree of medical sophistication equated cancer with death. It's amazing how the word *cancer* got our attention and made our lives, and the realization of their fragility, a piercingly urgent priority. Everything else simply stopped for us.

Although it was often out of character, we coped with the shock of diagnosis by crying, either immediately or later, when we fully realized the significance of the news.

Daria started crying when she heard the news in the hospital and left as quickly as she could "because I didn't want to be seen crying in the facility where I work." She spent the whole day at home sobbing hysterically. She says, "That's not my style, but it sure happened that day." Betsy also cried off and on for the first two days. She says, "Nothing else in my life mattered. All I could do was cry."

Some of us had a delayed reaction. Joy did not experience her emotions until the day she returned home from the hospital following her mastectomy. She says that after her mastectomy she felt completely in control, but that she wasn't dealing with her diagnosis, just taking care of business, "doing everything in an orderly fashion, making out lists, checking things off. I handled my breast cancer as if I were putting together a real estate transaction. You cover the bases, you present the offer. That's the way I felt." But on the day she came home from the hospital, she walked toward her bedroom and caught sight of herself in the mirror at the end of the hall. "When I looked in the mirror, I saw my seventy-year-old mother the way she'd looked when she stayed with me right after she had surgery to save her leg because of her diabetes. She died of a stroke shortly after. She was very ill at the end and looked so unkempt. I saw my mother, who was always so dependent on everybody else, totally unable to cope with anything. All at once I realized that I was a different person now, I wasn't the same woman who had checked into the hospital a week before. That was the first time I cried. I went into my bedroom and closed the door and sobbed until I made myself sick."

Carol S. explains that she has yet to cry hard about her diagnosis of breast cancer. "I still haven't cried since the few tears I shed just after hearing the diagnosis. I'm sure

> Secondary victimization, or downward comparison, occurs when events, such as a diagnosis of breast cancer, threaten a person's self-esteem and social valuation. The patient is able to feel better about her situation by comparing it to someone whose condition is worse. This comparison is usually done in the early stages of adaptation to the illness.
>
> Hagopian, G. "Cognitive Strategies Used in Adapting to a Cancer Diagnosis." *Oncology Nursing Forum.* 20(5) (1993): 759–63.

that one day all of this will sink in and I will have to come to terms with my emotions. But that hasn't happened yet. Maybe I still haven't accepted the diagnosis."

In addition to the emotional release of crying, we coped with the emotions evoked by our diagnosis by using a strategy that psychologists call downward comparison, that is, comparing our situation with situations we perceive to be worse.

Daria explains, "Late in the evening of my diagnosis, after about six hours of sobbing, I said to myself, Okay, it's time to process. Define the problem. Think it through. I decided that if God had told me I was going to get cancer and I could pick the type, I would have chosen breast cancer over all other malignancies. I can cut off my breasts and have a good chance of ridding myself of the cancer. It's not cancer of the colon requiring a colostomy. It's not cancer of the brain involving loss of the ability to think clearly and make my own decisions. It's not a cancer that will cause me to lose half of my face. I also realized that having cancer myself was better than being given the burden of watching one of my children go through it. As soon as I went through the mental process of looking at the big picture, my self-control immediately returned. The next morning I was tearful but I wasn't hysterical. I was very much in control and able to function and start making decisions."

Most of us have experienced anger, periodically or continuously, since we received our diagnosis. Some of us are motivated by anger. We channel and harness it in order to drive ourselves to accomplish goals. Donna says, "People tell me to release this anger and anxiety. Well, that's nonsense. I need this energy and anxiety right now because I have very important decisions to make and I need this level of energy to be able to do what I need to do." Others of us believe that releasing our anger is critical so it will not harm us by causing stress and perhaps leading to further disease.

Our anger finds different targets. Donna has directed her rage "at a bad disease and an inadequate health-care system. I fault that health-care system for my misdiagnosis and for sometimes being insensitive and unkind to

According to some researchers, the way in which a cancer patient deals with her diagnosis may influence her prognosis. A study of sixty-nine breast cancer patients determined that patients who reacted to a diagnosis of cancer with denial or a fighting spirit demonstrated a higher rate of survival at five years after diagnosis than did those who reacted with stoic acceptance or helplessness/hopelessness.

Greer, S., Morris, T., Pettingale, K. W. "Psychological Response to Breast Cancer: Effect on Outcome." *The Lancet.* 2(8146) (Oct. 13, 1979):785–87.

women with breast cancer. The system makes you constantly struggle to maintain a leadership role. It is not a consumer-based business."

Sometimes our anger is hidden beneath the surface. Betsy says that she feels something is going on deep within herself, and she is "almost afraid to process it because my anger is so vast." Four years after her recurrence, Cathy says she still feels anger toward cancer that she usually is not aware of until it flares up. "Last year I lost a beloved dog to liver cancer. I was so angry that this damn disease could take something from me. He was an old dog and could have died from anything, but the fact that it was cancer made me furious. I didn't realize that I still had so much anger."

Carol H. believes that it required three battles with cancer before she was able to release her anger and prevent it from harming her again. "I had my first diagnosis, then a metastasis, then a second diagnosis, and I still wasn't ready to move through all the anger and resentment I'd held on to for so long. After fourteen years of dealing with and living every day with cancer, I decided I wasn't going to allow the emotions bottled up deep inside of me to hurt me again by causing more disease. It took me a long time to get to the point where I could release my anger and resentment not just against cancer, but also against lots of people and lots of events in my life. You don't let go of it until you are ready. It was a lot of work for me to change this behavior of mine that held feelings inside. I found I could let go of emotions only physically—I couldn't just process emotions in my head. I had to yell, scream, beat on the dashboard in the car, or hit a bed with a rolled-up towel. Once I released the guilt and anger, I didn't need or expect somebody else to make me number one. I did what I needed to be number one." She now walks four miles a day in the summer or does aerobics as a way to release her feelings and maintain peace and centeredness in her life. She says, "These lessons of letting go are powerful. Most of the time my life is so peaceful. It is just wonderful. But when the anger comes back and I feel I need to release it, I walk or do something really physical, such as beating my bed with a pillow."

Working Through Our Emotions

Some of us find that visualization techniques help us manage the anger and fear surrounding our breast cancer experience. While some experts recommend aggressive visualization techniques, such as seeing the cancer cells being devoured or destroyed, in general we prefer to use peaceful, loving images and to focus on loving our entire selves, cancer and all.

Techniques for emotional release:
- imagery and visualization
- journals
- exercising
- finding positive examples
- support from family and friends
- prayer and meditation

Joy observes, "I tried those images of various things destroying the cancer cells, but I couldn't deal with the violence. To me, the cancer cells were a part of my body, so they could not totally be an enemy." Instead she developed a visualization technique that involves mentally placing her worries and problems on individual leaves, then watching the leaves fall from the tree into a lake and drift away. She says, "I mentally put a problem I'm worrying about on a leaf and watch it disappear. It allows me to let go of my worries and fears. You can't imagine the peace it brings me."

Cathy kept an audio journal of her feelings after she was diagnosed the second time and went through surgery and reconstruction. Many of us continue to rely on exercise to work through our feelings of distress and frustration. It has also been very important for us to find and talk with other women who have experienced breast cancer and who now are active, vital, and positive about their futures.

For all of us, the support of our family and friends has been an invaluable source of stability and refuge, even though we continue to worry about how they are handling our disease. We all believe we are lucky to have people close to us who allow us to express our true feelings when they become too much to handle alone.

Support Groups

Approximately half of us find peace and emotional encouragement by participating in support groups. Some of us joined support groups following our primary diagnosis, while others did not become involved until we experienced recurrence or metastasis.

Sally chose not to join a support group following her primary diagnosis, but she became involved when her breast cancer metastasized. "When I got the diagnosis of my metastasis, all of a sudden cancer was interrupting my life, and I decided I would go to the support group. I hate to miss a meeting now. The group has been so important to me."

Others of us have found different means of meeting our emotional needs. Donna explains, "When I was first diagnosed, I felt that as a nurse I already knew a lot about breast cancer. I didn't feel that I had enough energy to take care of myself and to support other women in a group. Also, my perception then was that I didn't want to be with women in the advanced stages of breast cancer. I thought it would just drag me down, and I was all about going on with my life and living it to the fullest. Besides, my husband is wonderfully supportive, and we leaned on each other."

Each of us has had different experiences, positive and negative, with support groups. Our reactions depended largely on our own needs and desires and the chemistry between us and a particular group or leader. Those who have found support groups invaluable believe that the key to success is finding a group that provides a good match with your emotional needs and personality.

Finding the right support group:

- participant mix (type of cancer, stage, primary, recurrent, etc.)
- philosophy and objectives of the facilitator
- flexibility regarding commitment to participation

Comfort Level

Cathy says, "Choosing a support group is like choosing any other part of your breast cancer team. The most important thing is that you feel comfortable with them. A particular support group can be right for one woman and wrong for another. You just have to go and see how you feel there. I do think you should give a support group a fair chance by attending at least a couple of times, unless your first visit is a total disaster."

Support groups have different personalities, depending on their objectives, members, leader(s), structure, and focus. The tone or focus of a particular group may make you uncomfortable. For example, Donna objected to the emphasis one support group facilitator placed on the belief that women with breast cancer created the cancer themselves by leading a stressful life.

Cathy attended a lumpectomy support group but found that she could not identify with the other women: "It was a small group, and most of the women expressed a lot of anger toward the medical establishment and toward men in general. Their anger became a major focus of the discussions. I couldn't identify with them—that isn't how I view my breast cancer experience, so I left the group."

Group Flexibility

Carol S. first attended a support group that allowed women to drop in rather than become committed members: "I went two or three times and found different people at each meeting. I wanted more continuity, so I found an ongoing group sponsored by one of the local hospitals. We have a fairly stable core of women, and that feels right for me."

Group Composition

The composition of the support group is another factor to consider. Some groups are open to both men and women with any type of cancer, while others limit participation to individuals with a specific type of cancer, such as women with breast cancer. Some women benefit from attending a mixed group because they appreciate that breast cancer is more treatable and curable than many other cancers. However, support groups composed solely of women with breast cancer can offer more specific information and insight. Some support groups are fairly homogeneous, that is, they allow only women with a certain stage of breast cancer, while others accept women with all stages of the disease.

There are advantages and disadvantages to mixing women with different stages of breast cancer. Some women with Stage I breast cancer may find it upsetting or depressing to belong to a support group including women in later stages of the disease or women who have metastatic disease. Others may feel they can benefit from the experience of those further along in the disease.

Advantages of a support group:

- specific information and insight
- inspiration
- opportunities to contribute what you've learned
- being with those who understand your fears and anxieties
- relieves burden from family and friends who cannot empathize because they have not experienced the disease

Advantages

Women in support groups are an invaluable source of firsthand information about the reality of undergoing treatments such as surgery, chemotherapy, and radiation.

Several of us consulted women in support groups when we were in the process of choosing therapeutic options.

Those of us who are involved in support groups find that one of the primary benefits is being with other women with breast cancer—women who can validate our feelings, understand our fears and anxieties, and provide us with information. We believe that support groups allow us to share our experiences, strengths, and hopes in an atmosphere that is safe and honest.

Sally says, "It's amazing the support we give one another, even though we seldom contact each other outside of the group. It's a place where you can talk about what you are feeling and what you are experiencing, and the others understand. People who haven't had breast cancer will try to give advice or try to be encouraging, but they haven't been there. We have all been very encouraged, too, about the studies showing that women with breast cancer who participate in support groups tend to live longer."

The women in our support groups also provide us with positive examples. Betsy says, "Two years after my treatment, I'm still meeting my support group for dinner every month or so. The board of the Breast Cancer Coalition meets almost every month, and I've seen several members diagnosed with metastatic disease, and it is hard watching them endure further treatment. But they are back at the next board meeting advocating change. One of our members died, and we watched her die. She was very brave and full of a sense of humor. A month before her death, she got on a bus with us and went to Washington and met with President and Mrs. Clinton. I said to myself, "Man, what a role model." That's the kind of person I want and need to see. And I want to see people like Joy who have courageously fought recurrence and metastases

A now-famous study conducted by Spiegel, et al. determined that psychosocial intervention, in the form of support groups, has a positive effect on survival for patients with metastatic breast cancer. Eighty-six women were randomized to receive either one year of weekly support group therapy, self-hypnosis for pain management and their regular oncologic treatment, or only routine oncologic treatment. Survival time for patients receiving the support group treatment had an overall survival time of 36.6 months from time of randomization as compared with the control group's survival time of 18.9 months. The effect of treatment on longevity was not apparent until about eight months after the study ended.

Participants underwent a battery of psychological tests prior to the study, none of which determined any significant psychological differences among patients. This study was undertaken to determine the role that psychological support has on anxiety, depression, and pain, without affecting the course of the disease. The researchers wanted to disprove the claims that the right mind-set can conquer cancer. Spiegel and associates were surprised to find that psychosocial intervention had a tremendous impact on survival.

Spiegel, D., Bloom, J., Kraemer, H. C., et al. "Effect of Psychosocial Treatment on Survival of Patients with Metastatic Breast Cancer." *The Lancet.* 2(8668) (Oct. 14, 1989):888–91.

and who have wonderful stories and are wonderful role models. I can look to these women and say, 'God, that's great! That's how it should be done.'"

Participating in support groups also gives us the opportunity to help other women with breast cancer. Sally explains, "The women in our group are decision makers. A lot of times women come who are not as skilled at making decisions, and they've simply agreed to whatever their physician recommended. One young mother of a two-year-old and a four-year-old was upset because her surgery was scheduled for the next week and she hadn't had time to prepare for it and she wasn't sure it was the right option for her. We told her she was in charge and she didn't have to have that operation the next week or go along with recommendations that she didn't feel were best for her. We show women that they can exercise control. After talking with us, a lot of women seek a second opinion, find another physician, or change their treatment plan. We act as advocates for every woman in our support group. It's an important role, and we believe we're helping women get the best possible care and make the best decisions."

None of us has chosen participation in a support group to the exclusion of individual support from family, partners, and friends. Instead of taking the place of relationships with our families and friends, support groups provide a different kind of comfort. We often find it easier to discuss our fears and feelings regarding breast cancer with women in a support group because we worry about upsetting or causing anxiety for those who love us. We do not have to consider whether the women in our support groups are tired of hearing us talk about breast cancer, or whether they will become impatient with our fears if we repeat them too often. Finally, no matter how much our family and friends try to understand our situations, they have not traveled along the same path.

Betsy explains, "When I want to talk about breast cancer, I talk to my support group, to women I know who have had breast cancer. I have confidence in them and know they will listen to my story. It's not that my family isn't supportive. They are. They love me. But what I've fi-

Fawzy et al. evaluated the immediate and long-term effect of psychosocial support on the immune system. Sixty-one patients were randomized to receive either six weeks of structured psychiatric intervention as well as routine treatment for melanoma (n=35) or routine treatment only (n=26). The group receiving interventions demonstrated reduced levels of distress, better coping methods, as well as significantly higher levels of immune response. Natural killer cells (NK) and other helper cells that are normally repressed during cancer were significantly elevated at both six weeks and six months after the psychiatric intervention. Psychosocial support seems to have physical as well as emotional benefits.

Fawzy, F., Kemeny, M., Fawzy, N., et al. "A Structured Psychiatric Intervention for Cancer Patients." *Archives of General Psychiatry.* 47 (1990):729–35.

nally figured out is that my family wants my breast cancer to be behind us. They don't want to hear that I'm still scared, that I worry about it recurring. They don't want to hear me talking about drawing up my will. They want me to be all right. They want it to be over. Period. And so the only people I can talk to about my fears are other women who've had breast cancer. They understand. I can say to them, 'I have a crick in my neck, do you think it's bone cancer?' and they'll talk to me about it; they won't fall apart."

Carol S. says, "I go to my support group, and breast cancer is all we talk about, and I find this a tremendous relief. We don't have to apologize about cancer. We don't have to tiptoe around feelings. It is so different from talking with my friends, even my closest friends."

Cathy agrees that support groups meet different needs. "It's wonderful to talk to the women in a support group and not have to preface everything with 'I know this sounds ridiculous but' . . . I can say, 'My shoulder is hurting and I'm afraid it's bone cancer,' and everyone in the room understands; they've felt the same way. It's a wonderful relief not to have to worry about people misinterpreting what you say. When a breast cancer survivor asks, 'Cathy, how are you doing?' I know she really understands where I'm coming from. I don't have to say, 'I'm doing fine.' I can cut right through and talk about how I really am doing. I can't do that with most other people, not even my family."

The Fear of Recurrence

Each of us has to live with the fear that our cancer will recur or metastasize, and for some of us, this fear has become a reality. We understand that there are no guarantees. If someone could give us a formula for never having cancer again, we would follow it, but no one can. As Betsy says, "We just have to live with the uncertainty."

As Daria explains, the uncertainty is always present. "It has been a year since my diagnosis, and I feel fortunate, but I never feel absolutely confident that I'm disease-free. I wouldn't be all that surprised if cancer popped up again. I don't know what corner it's going to be around. If I knew that it would come back in five years, I could plan the time and fit in everything I want to do. But I don't know. It's a big question mark. I figure, just wait and see what happens. I figure another Christmas, another whatever, that would be great, one more year."

The fear of recurrence ranks among the major issues for cancer survivors. A study of forty cancer patients with malignancies found that, in moderation, this fear may be beneficial in adapting to recurrence. Patients who reported an awareness of the risk of recurrence were less likely to suffer from intrusive stress symptoms when the recurrence actually occurred. Those patients who felt confident that they were cured of cancer were at the highest risk for developing intrusive stress response after recurrence. Patients who expected a recurrence faired poorly also.

In this study patients universally reported that recurrence was much more upsetting than the initial diagnosis. Patients reported less support from family and friends, and less information and support provided by the health-care team. All but one patient in the study reported that the recurrence had a far more damaging impact on their sense of hope than had the initial diagnosis.

Cella, D. F., Mahon, S. M., Donovan, M. F. "Cancer Recurrence as a Traumatic Event." *Behavioral Medicine.* 16(1) (Spring 1990):15–22.

We have all found ways to manage our fear of recurrence and metastasis. Carol W. says, "I can't change the fact that I have contracted this disease. There is nothing I can do except hope and pray that it won't come back again, but if it does, I'll be able to handle it and do what it takes so that it won't control me. I don't belabor it and wear myself out thinking about the disease. I let it alone."

Those of us who had recurrences or metastases experienced a different emotional response with the second diagnosis.

Recurrence—a totally different experience:

- there are no guarantees
- start over, reeducate yourself, and face the inconveniences of the medical system
- your risk of disability/death is significantly increased
- this realization adds a dimension to your emotional adjustment
- expect an even stronger proactive response because recurrence tends to add focus to your efforts

Cathy explains, "I do think the emotional response to recurrence is totally different. After the first time, I had put breast cancer behind me. I caught it early, had a lumpectomy, follow-up radiation, and I went on with my life. It's not that I thought the cancer would never come back, but I was diligent about my breast self-exams, mammograms, and everything else. I had closed that chapter, and when the same book hit me in the face again, I was stunned. The emotions were different from the first time. It was really scary to think that all the things I'd done hadn't worked, and the cancer was back inside me. I started making calls and gathering research right away, even before I had confirmation of the recurrence. I felt just as ignorant as the first time. Like 'Gosh, I don't know anything about mastectomy. Now I have to start all over.' It was much harder on me to hear that diagnosis the second time. It was very hard."

When the physician gave her the diagnosis of another metastasis of her breast cancer, Joy told herself, "Let's just get out the back door—don't let anybody see you because, Joy, you're going to lose it this time. This time you're going to lose it, . . . the cancer just can't have come back again. You can't muster what it takes to go through chemotherapy and radiation again. There's no way you've got the energy to get through it."

Donna describes how her reaction to the news that her disease had metastasized differed from her reaction to her primary diagnosis. "With my initial diagnosis, my emotional reaction was fear, sadness, and isolation. I thought, What a horrible, devastating experience this is. This is big. This is scary. I was stunned. I cried. Since I got the diagnosis of metastatic disease—it's hard to believe—but I've only spent perhaps one day feeling sad. Instead I'm overcome, not with anger, but with rage. I look back on my thirty-nine years and I'm not sure that I've ever been really angry. I'm angry now. Once you get metastatic disease, you hear, 'Well, we just don't know.' And I say, 'Don't give me this bullshit that you don't know. Your not knowing means I may die.'"

Disability and Death

We also live with the fear of disability and death. We find that accepting death as a possible outcome of our disease is less difficult than coping with the prospect of disability and not being able to control the circumstances of our death. Sally explains, "I have thought a lot about death and have discovered I'm not afraid of dying. When the time comes, I'm willing. I am not afraid of the dying process." Joy echoes that sentiment. "I'm not afraid of dying, but I want to do it with dignity."

Each of us has thought about death, and we have each come to terms with it on a very personal level. Our major concerns are disability, dignity, pain, the possible inability to function normally, and our families. It is sad and difficult to contemplate our own deaths, especially to imagine how those we love, and who love us, will take it. We know these issues require a lot of thought, but we believe it is important to think them through, even now, even if you have just received your diagnosis. It is important to carefully consider how to make things right for you and your family.

Our greatest concern is quality of life, and we fear the loss of our ability to function normally. As women who have always been in control and who have taken care of others, we do not want to become dependent upon our families and friends. Some of us have watched terminally ill relatives and friends suffer for months and years before they died, and we do not want our families to be subjected to a similar experience with us. We also fear the pain that can accompany the final stages of breast cancer, and although there are pain medications available, we wonder about our alertness and ability to function while on these medications.

Some of us have considered euthanasia as a means of dying with dignity and in the manner we choose. As one of us reflects, "I will not go through tremendous suffering and pain if I have a choice. I will not waste away to nothing if I have a choice." Another says, "It is better to plan your death so that you have a chance to say good-bye and die in a beautiful way surrounded by the people you choose instead of being in some hospital room, hooked up to machines, and dying in the middle of the night with no one there."

Reflections on dying:

- dying with dignity

- controlling the dying process
- making sure your family is aware of your decision
- being able to discuss this openly with spouse/partner and family
- saying all that needs to be said before it is too late
- having someone close to you at the time of death

Others of us are opposed to the idea of engineering our own deaths, primarily because of our own or our family's religious beliefs. We have, however, come to terms with how we would proceed. "The truth of the matter is very clear—this is not a decision that anyone can make for anyone else, and it is a fantasy until it becomes real."

Cancer as a Wake-Up Call

*"I realized that I had been given a wake-up call, not a
call to death."*
—*Carol Hebestreit*

We are all in high-stress professions, and we all love our
work. But the diagnosis of breast cancer has forced us to
examine what our work really means in our lives and to
our health. Work-related stress is usually portrayed as a
negative aspect of a person's life, but for most of us it is
the thing on which we thrive. It is exhausting, and it is invigorating—the thrill of the performance and the accomplishment. Stress is like a drug—addictive and harmful—
unless used in moderation.

The Impact of Stress

We do not believe that women should blame themselves
for developing breast cancer. Yet we wonder if stress may
have played a role in the development of our breast cancers. Many of us had experienced years of chronic stress
caused by working long hours, being single parents and
sole income producers, assuming responsibility for many

people in our lives both at work and at home, and simply "piling too much on our plates." Like most newly diagnosed cancer patients, many of us can also point to a period of unusually severe stress shortly before our diagnosis. For example, in the three years preceding her primary breast cancer, Sally experienced her mother's death; a divorce; the loss of her job; and a move and a new job in another part of the country, far from family and friends. Daria believes the lump in her breast grew as rapidly as it did because of an extremely stressful situation at work. During the eighteen months before her diagnosis, Betsy had closed a law practice of fifteen years and moved from New Orleans to New York City. Carol H. found the lump in her breast nine months after her sister died of AIDS after years of misdiagnosis because she did not fit the medical model of the "typical" HIV patient. Donna's dad died nine months before her diagnosis. After years as a single parent, Joy had married a kind and thoughtful man who tragically became terminally ill shortly thereafter. She had to cope with his failing health and the severe personality changes that resulted from his illness. She also had to continue to care for her family as well as produce as much or more volume than ever in her real estate business. She needed to prepare for the possibility of assuming a tremendous financial burden as a result of both her husband's disease progression and that she would once again assume total financial responsibility for her two teenage daughters.

Breast cancer develops as a result of a complex web of genetic, environmental, constitutional, and other factors that researchers have not yet been able to unravel. Although we know intellectually that no woman can lead her life in a way that guarantees she will not develop breast cancer, it is difficult for some of us not to feel at

Cooper et al. explored the relationship between psychosocial stress and the incidence of breast cancer in 1,956 women attending breast screening clinics in England. The women were compared with 567 control subjects attending a well-woman clinic also in England. Subjects were asked to complete a life-events questionnaire prior to diagnosis. The women were then divided into four groups: those with normal breasts, those with benign results, those with cysts, and those with cancer. The researchers determined that the death of a patient's husband, family member, or close personal friend is frequently associated with the diagnosis of breast cancer. Personal illness was also determined to be associated with a diagnosis of breast cancer, particularly if the illness involved surgery or hospitalization. Recent termination of employment and retirement were also more common in the breast cancer group than in the other groups.

One surprising finding was that, irrespective of the incidence of any given life-event, the cancer group perceived it as being more severe than the cyst group, who perceived stress as being more severe than the benign or normal groups. Researchers noted that the greater the perceived impact of any given life-event, the greater the risk of breast cancer and the greater the severity of the disease.

Cooper, C. L., Cooper, R., Faragher, E. B. "Incidence and Perception of Psychosocial Stress: The Relationship with Breast Cancer." *Psychological Medicine*. 19 (1989):415–22.

least partly responsible for our disease. Carol H. explains, "Being a controller makes you feel even worse when you get cancer because you think you must have had something to do with it." Betsy questioned whether her persistent level of stress played a role in the develop-

ment of her breast cancer. "I wanted to do it all and I did.
I'd had my foot on the pedal for years, and when I was
diagnosed, I thought it was payback time. I felt some responsibility because I hadn't been prudent in terms of my
lifestyle and watching my health."

All of us agree that the diagnosis of cancer made us
slow down and reevaluate the way we were living our
lives—something we had been intending to do for years.
Daria says, "I knew that I needed to slow down, but the
nature of my work wouldn't allow me to. When I was diagnosed with breast cancer, I felt as if someone said,
'Okay, sweetheart, you won't slow down? Bam, deal with
this—cancer will force you to change.'"

Sally did not truly change her lifestyle until her cancer
metastasized. "The first time around, I interpreted cancer
as a warning, and I changed my attitude about life. When
I thought I was cured, I fell right back into the same old
grind. Then the metastasis came. I felt as if the Lord had
to take another big board and hit me across the side of
my head to get my attention. This time I listened."

We had to assess:

- our commitment to our careers
- the nature of our work
- the level of stress in our lives
- our sense of responsibility to others
- the value of time and money

Breast cancer forced us to take a fresh look at our commitment to our careers, the nature of our work, the level
of stress in our lives, and the sense of responsibility we
feel for other people. Living with medical uncertainty
caused us to view both time and money differently. We re-

defined our priorities regarding ourselves, our ambitions, our political commitments, and our personal relationships. We became more self-focused. We wanted more time in both our professional and our personal lives to do the things we truly enjoy. We want to control how we will spend the next twenty years. Most of all, we did not, and do not, want to waste a single moment.

After Amy left the world of finance, she opened her own consulting business before joining NABCO. One of her objectives was to have a flexible work schedule that would allow her time for two new priorities: meeting new friends (and hopefully a new romance) and volunteering in a breast cancer organization. She relates that "volunteering was extremely important to me, verging on the crucial. As many people do, I had a sense that I had been fortunate with my breast cancer diagnosis. It had been detected early by sheer luck. I had access to and could afford the best medical care in New York City, although I was amazed to find how little was known about the disease and how best to treat it. . . . Thinking back, I know I subconsciously forged a deal of sorts with fate, something like 'I'll put my intellect and experience to work on breast cancer, as long as you make me safe.' I had read about the National Alliance of Breast Cancer Organizations and began at NABCO as a volunteer in 1987."

Cathy says that her recurrence caused her to "reevaluate everything and everyone." Carol H. explains, "I realized that God had given me a wake-up call, not a call to death. I decided to take a good look at my entire life, to examine my behavior, and to ask what do I need to change?" Sally realized that she had always lived her life for the future, saving money for a later date, waiting to meet the right man, or delaying travel until she had time. Her experience with cancer taught her to live in the present because the future is so uncertain.

Work and Money

Many of us no longer place the same value on money that we did before our diagnoses. Although we are concerned about meeting our financial responsibilities to others, we now view money as a commodity that is necessary for living, not as an indicator of our success. For example, Joy decided that she was no longer willing to work twenty hours a day to maintain her level of income. She reduced her sales volume, which had ranged from between seven and ten million dollars, to about three million dollars a year.

Breast cancer allowed Daria to choose not to continue working at the same pace. "Cancer has helped me say 'enough is enough.' Originally my plan was to work incredible hours until I was fifty, make a lot of money, then retire early. Now I realize that I might not see age fifty. My professional life is important to me and I enjoy health care, but I don't want to kill myself doing it. I cherish my time off, and I'm committed now to having more of it, which may involve a career shift from my present responsibilities. I'm not sure where my career will be in five years."

In addition to reconsidering our level of income, some of us changed the focus of our jobs to derive more satisfaction from our work. Joy switched from concentrating on the high end of the housing market to working with first-time home buyers. She enjoys assisting young people who are just starting out in life and accepts the fact that she has to sell more houses to earn the same income. Betsy practices law in different areas, including some medical law. She represents some women with breast cancer who were misdiagnosed or treated inappropriately.

Cathy explains how breast cancer changed her work. "Now I have a mission—to save lives by using television to educate women about breast cancer. I work longer and harder than I did before—I practically live in the office. The difference is that the work I am doing is more meaningful and I now delegate tasks that I don't enjoy to other people. I always felt it was easier to do something myself than to try to get somebody else to do it. Now I make time to do the creative part of my job, the part I like the best."

Reordering our priorities and changing our career goals was, and is, a complex undertaking. Carol S. would prefer to devote more time to research, writing, and political advocacy and less to teaching and holding administrative positions in the academic world. Yet she must consider that changing her ambitions affects her ability to financially assist her mother and her son. She also feels that because her generation is the first to reach the upper levels of academic institutions, she has a responsibility to younger women to strive for a top position in a university. She recognizes that she may have to trust others to carry on. "I may have to miss out on this one. But I also believe that by passing on some of the commitments, causes, and options, I may be able to create new opportunities I hadn't even anticipated."

Donna feels that her work is an important part of who she is, and she wants to maintain a balance between her personal and professional lives for as long as possible. At the same time, she wants to travel around the world with her husband and do other things that will require relinquishing her job and accepting the possibility that it might not be available to her when she wants to return to work.

Personal Responsibilities

Many of us were accustomed to being responsible for our children, our parents, and other members of our families in addition to our professional responsibilities. Our diagnoses of breast cancer caused us to reevaluate our sense of responsibility and, when it was appropriate, to let go. Carol H. explains, "Until my cancer metastasized, I was giving out one hundred percent of Carol to everyone. I was a caretaker for my children, my family, people I worked with—you name it. I decided it was time to reexamine my control issues and caretaking issues, and to focus on myself. It has changed my perspective on how long I want to work and what I want to do with the time I have left."

When her physicians told her that she was terminally ill, Joy realized that her grown children needed to start taking care of themselves because she might not be around to care for them. Carol W. recalls that she told her brothers, "'Guess what, after all of these years of taking care of you, I am not your mother.' I made a concerted effort to change some of the responsibilities that I'd allowed myself to take on. I stopped saying, 'Sure, pile everything on me.' It represents a major change in my life since my diagnosis."

Our Priorities and Professional Style

The experience of having cancer has also made us attempt to change our behavior and personalities. We try, though often unsuccessfully, to exhibit less driving, aggressive behavior. We are learning to be more patient, more mellow, more forgiving, and to pay less attention to other people's expectations of us. We have tried to resolve our differences with people in order to reduce the problems in our lives. Betsy says her effort to be "nicer" lasted about twenty minutes, but she at least made the effort! Carol W. explains, "I have cleaned up a lot of the muck and mire that was a part of my life prior to my diagnosis. I want to be able to deal with this disease without being hindered by unfinished business."

We are slowly but surely learning to say no to activities and responsibilities that we do not enjoy, and we are allocating time for things we want to do. Carol W. says, "Before my diagnosis, I always said, 'I'll do that later'— whether it was taking a vacation or catching a movie. Now I think it's time for me to be a bit more selfish and do what Carol wants to do." We are becoming more protective of our time because we feel that, in one sense, time is all we have. Sally says, "It has been difficult for me to learn to control the way I spend my time because I've always tried to please other people. Now I've learned that I can tell people what my needs are, and they usually respect that."

We are learning to establish boundaries and to protect our need for time and space for ourselves. Carol S. says, "When the news of my diagnosis got around, I had houseguests several weekends in a row. All my friends and relatives wanted to come and see how I was, to let me know they were concerned. It took a long time for me to be able to say, 'It's too much. I don't want you to come.' A close friend was going to come visit with her husband and her two young kids. And I told her, 'I really want to see you, but I don't want the whole family. If you can come alone, fine.' I'm finally learning to put my own needs first—at least part of the time."

Our View of Time

Our experience with breast cancer has left us with a different sense of time. At first we experienced a sense of urgency that has been somewhat moderated as time passes. It is difficult to maintain a feeling of urgency and desperation. It passes and "normalcy" returns as we begin to believe that maybe we will be around next month, next year. We have learned to adjust the way we plan. A good model for us is Joy. After dealing with cancer for nine years, she has changed her planning horizon and no longer makes five- and ten-year goals for herself. She establishes minigoals instead, using timelines of three or six months.

We still feel a need to make time work for us. We have tried to take assertive steps to make things happen according to our schedule. We try to move things along at work. Now is important; we want to get things done because if "it" comes back it may be too late. We struggle with prioritizing, especially when we have to choose between our personal and professional plans, asking ourselves, What comes first? Work, time for myself, time for my family, time to do things I've always wanted to do?

It is a difficult struggle. We find ourselves trying to put everything "first." We want to hurry everything along. A heightened sense of our own place in our orchestrated scheme will be our salvation. We are teaching ourselves that we are the central figure in our plans.

Putting Ourselves First

We realize, however, that in many cases, putting ourselves first is not practical. We still hurry to meet deadlines, to catch a plane, to catch up. None of us wants to become the "professional breast cancer patient." We already have professions. This inability to slow down is probably innate and is sometimes difficult to integrate with a careful approach to daily life. Betsy explains, "I want to do everything now. My secretary and my colleagues must think I'm a prima donna when I say to them, 'Don't you understand? We have to do this now!' I refuse to lose a minute because if I get sick again, I may be disabled. If something isn't right, even if it's just a hotel room, I want to move on—I can't waste time."

Sally expresses the same sentiment. "I'm driven to spend every moment happily and actively because I don't know how much time is left. I hope that I have another twenty years, but it may only be two or three or five years. In my support group, we constantly talk about how lucky we are to have learned to live fully in the present. We regret that we had to get cancer to learn that lesson. We wish we could get the word out to people so they won't have to experience cancer in order to understand that every moment is precious."

We're Changing—Slowly

We have also learned that we cannot change our old patterns of behavior overnight. No matter how strong our resolve to change, it is difficult to translate our good intentions into actions. We appreciate that leading our lives differently requires as much evolution as revolution. As a result, few of us have made the substantive changes one would expect following our experience with a life-threatening illness. Physical disability may be the only thing that slows us down.

Carol S. struggles to reduce her workload and find time to take care of herself. "My friends are worried because my pace hasn't changed. I'm booked from 7:30 A.M. until 11:00 P.M. day after day. I think my friends are right—I am tired and I need to do less. I want to unload instead of load up on things. It's an issue I've been dealing with forever. Cancer has made me be a little tougher, but it is difficult to change."

Betsy elaborates on the dilemma we all face when she explains, "I haven't been able to make substantial changes in my life. I still work sixty hours a week, but I spend forty practicing law and twenty doing breast cancer advocacy work. I like being a lawyer and an advocate, and I like the stress that goes along with it. My mind tells me I should stop doing all of this and devote my time exclusively to taking care of my health. But would it prolong my life? I'm torn. Part of me thinks I should go to Italy and live in a house by the sea. Another part of me knows that would last about five days and then I'd be organizing the whole town. I try to be realistic."

We have had to practice at satisfying ourselves rather than satisfying everyone else. Most of us are still learning this because it is hard to change focus—to place something else out front instead of our career or family. We started with little things like "Wouldn't it be great to travel?" or "I'd really like to get a little more sleep." What we have learned is that after lifetimes of putting our careers, our families, and our responsibilities first, we have to learn to put ourselves first; we need to find out what we want to do and do it. And, above all, we believe that what we are doing will be enough to keep breast cancer from killing us.

It Is as It Is—Yet More

"When you are diagnosed with breast cancer, you become an elder, no matter what your age. Through the events that occur, the decisions you make, the reevaluating and refocusing, you acquire wisdom and strength."

—Carol Stack

It goes without saying that we would never have chosen to have breast cancer. It has been utterly awful. Yet as we look back, we must admit that our "reluctant" journey has provided opportunities for personal growth that we might not have had otherwise. Surviving breast cancer has given us occasions to grow emotionally and spiritually, and it has taught us the value of our relationships with family, friends, and a higher power.

This experience can give you a stronger sense of:

- who you are
- what you can accomplish
- how you want to live your life
- the need to take better care of yourself

As breast cancer survivors, we have a stronger sense of who we are, of what we can accomplish, and of how we want to live our lives. We try to focus our attention on the present and to live each moment as fully as possible. We enjoy ourselves more than before because we have learned to listen to and respect our own needs, and we take better care of ourselves, both physically and emotionally. The simple fact that we have survived gives us a true sense of accomplishment.

Daria expresses how we feel about our experience: "I didn't choose breast cancer. Yet when I look back, at times when I'm not in the midst of heavy-duty emotions, I feel that breast cancer has changed me in a positive way. I'm sorry that I have to deal with it, but I also feel privileged. A lot of doors opened because of my breast cancer diagnosis and more are opening every single second."

Cathy explains that though she certainly would never say she is glad she developed breast cancer, she is happier today than before because through that experience she gained a clearer picture of who she is—and a purpose for her life and work. As she explains, "I understand now why I'm here. I'm here to help people." Sally believes that breast cancer has changed her life for the better in every

---

Although the journey is difficult, some women are able to move beyond the loss of a breast. The word *Amazon* comes from the words *a* (one) and *maza* (breast). To hunt more effectively with a bow and arrow, the fabled Amazons had a breast removed. Doing so was an important choice, which to them connoted enhanced ability.

Spiegel, D. "Conserving Breasts and Relationships." *Health Psychology*. 11(6) (1992):347–48.

> Spiegel theorizes that perhaps the loss of a breast and the subsequent turmoil and grief caused by the disease may be made up for in surprising ways. The enhanced support from friends and family, the reordering of priorities and relationships, and the discovery of what is of actual importance to each woman may add a new and surprisingly meaningful level to a woman's life.
>
> Spiegel, D. "Conserving Breasts and Relationships." *Health Psychology.* 11(6) (1992):347–48.

way. "My whole life has turned around. I've been happier these last three years than I ever was in my first forty years." Amy relates, "From a professional standpoint, this has been the most rewarding time of my life. . . . Businesswomen who have had breast cancer have a tremendous contribution to make to nonprofit organizations, as many of us are doing. In the process, we bring not only our expertise but also our personalities. It has been my experience that having breast cancer does not change the most basic skills—worriers still worry, procrastinators still stall, and workaholics still work too much. Even though I was working flat-out full-time for NABCO, it occurred to me that there was still a big job to do that no one was yet doing, and that was to mobilize survivors to political action."

For each of us, breast cancer was a catalyst for profound emotional and psychological growth. Joy sums up our feelings: "Today I am a very different woman from the woman who embarked on this battle with cancer nine years ago." The inner resources and strengths we were able to marshal to cope with the daunting and sometimes overwhelming challenge of breast cancer gave us a new sense of confidence. Cathy says, "I now feel that there is nothing I can't do, no challenge I can't handle. As much as I don't want to think about my cancer recurring, I know that I can do it again."

The experience of having breast cancer can be:

- a catalyst for emotional and psychological growth
- a means to gain practical knowledge
- an incentive to evaluate our professional priorities
- a way to bond with others in a unique sisterhood

Our breast cancer experience gave us practical knowledge, such as learning how to navigate the medical system. It also caused us to look at the world through different eyes and to feel wiser about life in general. Although we embarked on the journey reluctantly and before our time, breast cancer has served as a rite of passage for us. Carol S. says, "When you are diagnosed with breast cancer, you become an elder, no matter what your age. Through the events that occur, the decisions you make, the reevaluating and refocusing, you acquire wisdom and strength."

Our breast cancer journeys have given us a maturity and a feeling of inner calm that we had not known were possible. We have a stronger sense of who we are and of our potential. Carol W. explains that "I'm going to be me. I'm not going to waste time by being someone other than my true self. I'm much more vocal." Cathy says, "I live my life with a much clearer picture of who I am and of what I can accomplish. Having breast cancer pushed my career in a whole new direction and led to the most important and worthwhile contribution I've ever made—educating the public about breast cancer."

Being more confident of who we are, we have less desire to compete in order to prove our worth. As Joy says,
"Cancer made me realize that maybe it isn't necessary to
walk on water. Why does anyone want to walk on water
anyway?"

The breast cancer experience has also provided us with
a sense of belonging to a unique sisterhood. Cathy says,
"Like many professional women, I often felt that I didn't
fit in. At a very young age, I felt that there was nobody
quite like me, and maybe that's why I had such a strong
need to achieve. I now have a sense of belonging. I understand how my dad's generation can sit around and talk
about World War II for hours at a time. Exchanging war
stories with other breast cancer survivors validates my experience—we made it through the war."

The experience also has global dimensions in some of
our lives. Carol S. and a family in London traded graduate students. Charlotte, who was Peter and Elle's daughter, came to study at Berkeley and live with Carol. Carol's
son, Kevin, moved to England to study and acquired a
home away from home with Charlotte's parents. The two
families, who had not yet met, never anticipated the nature of the support that would come out of that ex-
change. Though thousands of miles away from home,
Kevin could count on Peter and Elle, who had herself
dealt with breast cancer, for affection and support when
he learned of his mother's cancer. Charlotte, on the other
hand, twice had to deal with cancer in loved ones, once
with her mother and a second time with Carol, her spir-
ited "adopted mom." Carol says, "Charlotte had a place
among the flowers in the garden; there she helped me
hold my face to the sun, and because of her humor, time
passed lightly." Coming full circle, Charlotte's mother

was once again in the midst of treatment before Charlotte returned home, and Kevin was there taking her place in his new "family." Both families spent Christmas in London together, and Carol says, "I found spunky new companions both in politics and in struggle."

A New Sense of Spirituality

Breast cancer has caused us to reevaluate our days, to search for the meaning in our lives, and to seek answers to difficult questions. We have come face-to-face with our mortality, and this has set us on a new, more spiritual path. At initial diagnosis, it was very important to maintain hope, to strive for a cure. This focus on cure as the elimination of disease fits nicely with our Western notion that illness and suffering are bad and that death is a catastrophe, a detestable state and not something to prepare for. Our culture cries out to cancer patients to "keep fighting." But, for some of us, the role of warrior, the metaphorical references to battles and fighting, just doesn't match our needs. In fact, for some of us who have metastatic and "incurable" disease, it seems strange to spend one's remaining days fighting an internal war.

By questioning our beliefs, we have heightened our sense of spirituality and now enjoy a new level of peace and acceptance. This peace and acceptance are most apparent in those of us who have had to deal with recurrence or metastasis. Carol H. has a glow about her whenever she speaks about her life, despite enduring first melanoma, then metastatic melanoma, and now breast cancer. She expresses her anger clearly and succinctly, though it is not so much about the cancer itself, but

rather about life's injustices. She feels freer now to discuss
the personal spiritual quest that has helped her attain this
level of acceptance.

Donna relates, "Since my metastasis, I've entered a
pensive, spiritual phase. I want to know why I'm here,
what I have contributed, and how my life fits into the
larger picture. I ask all sorts of questions. I go to the library to research other cultures and religions to find out
how they interpret life and spirituality. I have found much
in a book by Thomas Moore, called *Care of the Soul*, that
I understand and believe. I recognize that care of the soul
is not about curing, fixing, changing, but about the recognition that we have an absolute need for a spiritual life.
Many of us spend our lives avoiding anything unpleasant
and live a shallow life. Once I started opening to the pain,
I realized that much of what we feel is the emotional reaction, the fear, from our minds. For me, recognizing the
impermanence of this physical life was a revelation. That
doesn't mean I long for death; it means that I recognize
life and death are connected, an ongoing process that returns us to the source. My goal is to be healed, to be
whole. I want to let go of the anger so that love and compassion can surface. I want to be satisfied with who I am,
and not overly attached to this body. I am on a spiritual
journey, investigating more deeply every day."

Sally attributes her present level of joy and happiness to
the spiritual growth she has experienced since the diagnosis of her breast cancer. Following her primary diagnosis,
she found a church that matched her spiritual needs.
About the time her metastasis was diagnosed, she met her
significant other, Jim, which led to "the first decent relationship I've ever had in my life." Sally says, "I don't
think it's an accident that these things happened along
with my cancer—I believe my church was brought to me

because I was going to need it, and Jim was sent to me as a little angel to help me through."

Although she was a devout Christian before her primary diagnosis, breast cancer gave Cathy a much heightened sense of her relationship with God. She explains, "For me, religion was always a part of my life . . . but [I] had always positioned myself in leadership and teacher roles. I was always the one praying for other people . . . never the person in need, never the person asking others to pray for me. . . . I believed in the power of prayer. As such, I knew I would benefit from having others pray for me . . . to be the subject of others' prayers, rather than the one doing the praying. It felt awkward, uncomfortable, but I truly believe in the power of prayer . . . and I had to admit that, after people prayed for me (and many did), I felt better. From that time on, God became very real to me. Before, God was an idea. Today, God is so real to me that it's as if he's sitting right across the table. And I know now that he loves me as I am; that knowledge is a real blessing to me."

Joy says that her years of fighting cancer have allowed her to work through her beliefs about a higher power and to come to terms with the events of her life. This understanding has led her finally to peace and acceptance and has vanquished her fear of death.

We want to be cured. We hope that breast cancer will never again be a part of our lives. However, we acknowledge that there are stages of the disease when fighting is not necessarily the best option. In fact, a number of us have reacted negatively to suggestions from family, friends, and health-care professionals that we need to "fight" this disease in order to survive. Perhaps this term, used frequently by men, is one that is more acceptable to the male cancer patient. Many of us find it difficult to re-

A study of thirty recently diagnosed cancer patients determined that for the majority of these cancer patients, social support and faith were important factors in their journey through breast cancer. An interesting finding was that for 87 percent of these patients, formal religion was not an important factor in their lives. However, the majority felt that their faith in a supreme being was a constant and important factor. Many authors have noted that spirituality incorporates the quest to find meaning in life. This search for meaning seems to be both a spiritual and a psychosocial process.

O'Connor, A., Wicker, C., Germino, B. "Understanding the Cancer Patient's Search for Meaning." *Cancer Nursing.* 13(3) (1990):167–75.

late to the term and need to find other, more peaceful metaphors to help us reach the same objective. As Donna explains, "I don't want to imply that the answer to this disease is something as trivial as 'a fighting spirit.' ... I want to be healed, and *healed* has a totally different meaning from *cured*. Healed is being at peace with where I am now."

Enriched Personal Relationships

Our cancer has enhanced the intensity of our relationships with our partners, children, families, and friends. The challenges of dealing with a life-threatening illness have brought us closer, increased our respect for one another, and made us savor even the smallest moments together. Joy says, "The tiny things in life have become the big things as far as I'm concerned. The cancer experience

ing survivors of breast cancer to stand up for themselves and demand change. In 1991, she and other leaders of breast cancer advocacy groups cofounded the Breast Cancer Coalition to spearhead a grassroots movement to demand increased funding for breast cancer research; improved access to diagnosis and treatment for all women, especially the underserved and underinsured; and increased involvement and influence of breast cancer survivors in the medical and regulatory decisions that affect their lives. Amy says, "We began by stating the obvious: Women faced with a diagnosis of breast cancer find their lives turned upside down and become instantly consumed by the maze of treatment choices, medical decisions, and changes in their professional and personal lives. Navigating the maze is a challenge and, of necessity, a top priority. We felt that once women had made the decisions and were on their way to recovery, they would be ready to take the next step—to move past the personal dimensions of their disease to the political, to form a movement that could change the course of breast cancer. This was our way of fighting back in the face of grim facts that were making women angry then, and still are today."

Daria believes that perhaps one of the reasons the breast cancer experience was made a part of her life was to make her more effective in her profession. She wants to do the most she can with her experience. "I've been given this privilege, and I don't want to drop the ball. When newly diagnosed patients tell me they don't think they can deal with cancer, I can look them right in the eye and say, 'Yeah, I think you can deal with it because I did.' That helps a lot of people." Her experience as a patient enhanced her ability to be compassionate and understanding with her patients, especially those in particularly stressful situations in the emergency room.

Through the documentary about her breast cancer experience, Cathy reached more people than most of us could reach in a lifetime. She continues to produce segments related to breast cancer for *The Home Show*. She achieved her goal of airing one segment related to breast cancer on *The Home Show* each week during Breast Cancer Awareness Month. Three days after *The Home Show* publicized the National Breast Cancer Coalition's petition asking then presidential candidate Clinton to commit to increasing the funding for breast cancer research, an additional thirty-seven thousand people had signed the petition. She plans to continue educating the public. As she relates, "It has been four years since my recurrence and I keep saying, 'Okay, Lord, I'm ready for my next big project.' I hope it won't be cancer again, but I figure he knows best how I can help people. If I found out tomorrow that I have metastatic disease, I'd probably start thinking about how I could use that experience to help others. I'd probably go right to my producers and say, 'Here's a challenge for you. Do you want to help me share how to die?'" She also travels around the country to speak to groups about her experience.

All of us want to help other women deal with the terrifying possibility or reality of breast cancer. Carol W. trained as a group facilitator for SHARE, an organization devoted to education and advocacy for people with breast cancer. Though not currently active with SHARE, she will be working with the organization again in a few months. She says, "I have no problem standing up and talking about my experience. It's rewarding to hear someone respond, 'I'm glad that you spoke up because now I don't mind talking about what has happened to me.'" Daria is involved in lecturing during Breast Cancer Awareness Month and she tries to make it more than an ordinary lecture. Amy, as director of NABCO and as a member of the board of the National Breast Cancer Coalition, is a frequent speaker throughout the United States as well as other countries in which women are building groups for breast cancer education and advocacy. She also provides frequent testimony for congressional hearings dealing with breast cancer. Betsy volunteers twenty or more hours per week to the political activities of the National Breast Cancer Coalition, activities that have resulted in enormous increases in federal funding for breast cancer research. Joy does a breast cancer awareness program for realtors in the Portland area each year during Breast Cancer Awareness Month and has made a video for the Breast Center in Portland. She is also available on a referral basis to patients from the Breast Center as a role model for newly diagnosed women. Sally will be focusing her academic research in areas that pertain to breast cancer and the coping styles and psychological adaptations of women diagnosed with it.

As Amy says, "The jolt of diagnosis has made many of us see more clearly what is important, what we want, and maybe even how to get it. Often, our experience can help others. Incredibly, being a member of this club no one wanted to join has made our lives richer. Ultimately, that's what living is all about."

Having Faith and Hope

If we were to advise women on how to live with cancer, we would first urge them to find a place for the cancer in their lives and then put it away. Joy explains, "I restructured my will and took care of all those things, and then I went back to living. I don't make cancer my life." We

> Cancer is a crisis in the true meaning of the [word in] Chinese . . . , which is composed of two characters, one meaning *danger* and the other *opportunity*.
>
> Spiegel, D. "Conserving Breasts and Relationships." *Health Psychology.* 11(6) (1992):347–48.

would also counsel women to find a way to maintain their sense of humor no matter how grim the present moment is. As trite as it may sound, we believe that laughter is the best medicine. Most of all, we encourage women to remain hopeful.

Our advice to women with breast cancer:

- find a place for the cancer and then put it in its place
- remain hopeful
- maintain your sense of humor

Nine years ago, when Joy's physician informed her that she was terminally ill from breast cancer, she told him, "I may be terminal but I'm going to be long-term." She had two grandchildren when she was first diagnosed; she now has nine. Recently, for the first time in all her years of dealing with cancer, Joy's physician told her that he could use the word *remission.* Joy's experience proves that hope and expectation are not the same thing. Daria quotes an oncologist friend who said, "The medical expectation may be that you will not live another six months, but don't let that dash your hopes. When you buy a lottery ticket, do you expect to win or do you hope to win? Even if your probability of winning is only one in twenty thousand, someone is going to win, and it may be you." We all believe that Joy is the ultimate lottery winner; she has survived beyond all expectations. Sally agrees. "My physician said the stem-cell transplant gave me a 20 percent chance of surviving for two years. Well, my goal is to stay cancer-free for twenty years, and after twenty years, I'll renegotiate."

11

Till We Meet Again

Oᴜʀ sᴛᴏʀɪᴇs ᴄᴏɴᴛɪɴᴜᴇ, each along its individual and unique path. This chapter is about our meeting in May 1995, twenty months after this book begins, and about the subsequent events that have shaped our lives and moved us along those paths.

We had planned to meet in the late summer of 1995, and in our leisurely planning for that meeting, we considered what we would want to discuss. We anticipated moving from the vantage point of our first encounter, from which this book was created, to our lives as we are living them now.

Our busy schedules were already in high gear when we got the call that our reunion needed to be scheduled for the very next week. By that time, May 1995, Donna, who was one of the youngest among us at diagnosis and whose breast cancer journey started out hopeful, had rapidly moved into the very late stages of cancer.

We now prepared for the reunion with mixed feelings, under an umbrella of sorrow, knowing that we would likely be seeing one of our own for the last time. Despite this, we looked forward to seeing women with whom we had developed a close bond through our working together on this book. Donna particularly wanted this gathering to be a celebration of friendship, of our lives, and of *living*. Within weeks, Donna Cederberg, along with thousands of other women, would become part of the 1995 mortality statistics for deaths due to breast cancer.

Getting ourselves together with one week's notice was not an easy task. We dropped everything. Betsy canceled a business trip with her husband; Carol S. disregarded her book deadline; Cathy rescheduled television production meetings and found others to cover for her on a church committee; Joy canceled tickets for a trip to Holland; Sally missed the wedding of a close friend.

We consciously chose to be with Donna, and Donna chose to be with us. She was willing to take precious time from her life to hear about ours; to support us and to let us support her; to listen to our concerns and to talk about hers; and to let us all talk about the one subject we earnestly wanted to avoid—death and dying.

For two days of a beautiful southern spring, we met in Donna's hometown of Chapel Hill, at the Morehead House on the campus of the University of North Carolina. We juggled our emotions, stifled our tears, and focused on Donna, though she kept insisting that we should not do so. Special accommodations were needed for Donna and other members of the group living with daily pain; they were provided a place to rest between sessions. Like our first meeting, this one was videotaped to provide the basis for this chapter. Donna, elegantly buttressed with pillows in a chair, nudged us to talk about ourselves. We talked about our anger, disillusionment, exhaustion, and our sorrow. But most important, we were there to be with her. In the end, Donna's powerful presence and demeanor set us free to filter our own lives through her reality.

Donna moved back and forth between spirituality and humor, often seeming to be the host yet pushing us with her startling, rock-bottom honesty. "There's nothing magical about what I am doing right now. I am using the same skills I have always used," Donna told us as we joined her in this hastily arranged meeting so that we could be with someone we loved who was dying. At different times, each of us bit our lips trying to camouflage our well of tears. We were all together, but Donna had moved to the other side—she was dying. She was in a different place, experiencing what we all feared the most; and, at times, we could not help but express our admiration for her bravery.

Despite her pain and being heavily medicated, Donna zeroed in on our repressed feelings. There was such a passion inside her, which she wanted to add to this reunion. She had a lot to say; her very presence said so much—I'm here, be with me, listen to me, share with me; I'm not gone yet, I'm here. She reminded us of our bond of honesty and told us there were times she felt resentment toward friends who inferred that there was something magical about her. "It creates distance," she said. She was confident that when any of us progress to metastases (which Sally and Joy have already) and find ourselves facing death, that our coping skills would be there—"it's not a special, learned skill." Whatever we call it—magic, spirituality, self-awareness—Donna found that place that most of us search for all our lives, and she made it hers.

Settled in an elegant room in comfortable chairs, our two days of conversation took many turns. We spoke about what has changed for us and what has not, how we have grown personally and spiritually, what our fears are, and ultimately about facing death and dying. We did this with the honesty, caring, and humor that characterized our previous meeting.

The "Gift" of Cancer:
Our Personal and Spiritual Growth

It's hard to imagine that there is anything good that can come from having cancer, that there are gifts to be found in the experience. Yet we have all become stronger, more resilient because of it. Our "gifts" are unique, with each of us discovering our own. We talked a lot about what having cancer has meant in our lives.

For some of us, the growth was spiritual. This was often broader than religious growth and change. Donna said that "even though Mark and I are suffering, and it is the hardest time to pull out what is sacred inside of us, it can truly make a significant change in one's entire outlook on life." Donna and her husband, Mark, never referred to breast cancer as just Donna's disease. They talked about the treatment and the disease as "their" disease. They were in this together, from the very beginning.

Carol W. feels that having cancer deepened her spirituality and her relationship with God—strong faith is her enabler. As she told us, "I feel the meaning of my cancer has centered on my continued spiritual growth and the fact that, in this journey, I have learned the valuable lesson of 'to thine own self be true.' As my church-life expectations have increased, so has the biblical reminder that much is still required of me."

Sally confides that "I feel my cancer has provided me with an enhanced opportunity for spiritual growth. I am very active in my church when I am in Florida. I realize that I have little control over so many aspects of my life related to my breast cancer, but I have made the choice to live each day to its fullest, to love life in the way I have al-

ways done, and to be especially thankful for those days
when I am not in pain. My spiritual growth has meant a
great deal."

Cathy just completed three years of service as a deacon
in her church and has embarked on an intensive instructor's training course in advanced study of the Bible that
includes more than a two-year commitment and involves
a heavy course load. The work is hard, but she feels it has
already had a profound impact on her spiritual life. She
says, "Breast cancer is only one part of a spiritual journey
I have been on all my life. As frightened and unprepared
as I felt in that crisis, I can see now how God had prepared me for that challenge, and how I've grown and
'awakened' as a result of it. People who have experienced
cancer are among the most passionate, the most truly
alive people I know. We become acutely aware of our circumstances and feel the most alive when we are pushed
outside of our normal comfort zones—and cancer certainly pushes us into uncomfortable realms. I was never
more connected to God than when I was in crisis. Breast
cancer has served to reinforce my faith; I have a deeply
meaningful relationship with God and feel very clear
about what my spiritual beliefs are."

For Carol H., the journey has been a spiritual as well as
a physical one. As she says, "All my life I've been doing
and have never learned how to just *be*. I think that the experience of cancer has helped me to just *be,* which is so
different from *do*. It takes some time to learn to live and
be in the moment. Cancer taught me that I was not in control. This lesson proved to be valuable when I was put in
the position of having to resign from my job. I was able to
turn the situation into opportunity to 'learn to be.'"

"I have always been a confident person," Betsy says.
"Cancer has made me more so. I feel I am now more clear

about my priorities. I just don't get into responsibilities I don't want to."

"I have made the beginning of a lot of changes," Joy tells us. "I have learned I don't have to be a perfectionist. I have learned that I have not failed because I am not perfect."

"I have learned a lesson from cancer," Carol S. says. Carol had completed her most recent anthropological book, *Call to Home,* which was published three years after her initial diagnosis. "Perhaps this book, which meant so much to me, is done because I am more able and impassioned to set my own priorities—a task that hopelessly eluded me in the past." Carol and her mother have faced some difficult decisions together revolving around Carol's concern for the care of her mother, physically and financially. With Carol's mother now in a retirement home, Carol is free of her fears concerning her mother's financial future. "One gift I have received from illness," Carol says, "is that I now enjoy solitude and seek writing retreats for both serenity and clarity. I check my schedule still, but only to be sure that I am not burying my own priorities."

"Whenever I lay down to go to sleep," Daria says, "I think that this was a good day. Even on those rare days that I am sick, I feel good because if I'm dead I can't feel pain."

A Shift from Quantity to Quality of Life

We discovered that an overriding issue for all of us is our quality of life. Faced with our own mortality, we have made major adjustments in what we want and expect from our lives. Because we may be faced with less time, how we spend it becomes much more important.

Carol W. says, "I don't dwell on what might be coming because I am busy grappling with planning for the future, knowing it is more important to live each day to the fullest. Retirement is not in the 'as-planned schedule' anymore but is taking place sooner rather than later while there is yet healthy time. I look at the positive things now and take advantage of my strengths to keep me going forward."

Donna told us, "My time frame is daily now. I hope for a pain-free day. This day [at the reunion] is a big day for me. I will go home and crash. What we are trying not to do is think that this is the last time I will do this or anything else. We celebrate every day." As Donna stated, "Quality of life is very individual and can only be judged by the individual. Quality items for me are watching sunsets, enjoying wine, smelling good food, communing with Mark. . . . This time around, I deliberately chose not to take drugs with neurotoxicities. Where is the choice when there is no quality of life?"

As Betsy says, "Knowing the personality types we all are, we may still start at seven in the morning and end at eleven at night, but maybe we will be doing different things. It is an issue of time. I might still be checking my schedule; it may just be a different schedule."

"Making time to do things I enjoy—like travel—is important now," Cathy tells us. "Saving money for retirement is much lower on my agenda. The 'little things,' like giving and receiving hugs from people I love, have taken on new importance, too. When my recurrence was diagnosed, one friend at the office promised a 'hug a day' as his gift to my quality of life. It's been six years now, and we still do it."

"How did I get to this ten-year point?" Joy asks. "It's the quality of one's life, not the quantity. I have had some very beautiful times that no one will ever know about."

Finding Humor

Despite the crisis that caused our reunion to take place earlier than we had planned, humor was very much in evidence. We laughed at ourselves, and with each other. We find that humor is a necessary healing component of our everyday lives.

During our time together, Joy told us a particularly funny story about a man she dated. "At an amorous point," she related, "he put his hand on one of my breasts. I didn't notice what he was doing until he whispered that women my age generally didn't have such firm breasts, but he was certainly enjoying the experience. I told him I was glad he was getting pleasure from it because, as the result of my double mastectomy, they weren't my breasts and I couldn't feel a thing!"

Betsy tells us that her best coping style is humor. "I feel my ability to laugh at myself is probably the best approach I could have, whether I am telling a story about a vacation with my husband, my forgetfulness, or my day of insanity when I thought I might have bone metastasis."

Our Changing Appetites

Chemotherapy left long-lasting, perhaps permanent, changes, such as menopause, that affect the way we respond to food and to sex. Many of us found that not only our appetites for food were altered by chemotherapy but also our interest in, and desire for, sex. For some of us in relationships that were not strong enough, our diminished sex drive became a major obstacle. As a result, some of those relationships ended. For those of us who were in relationships that had stronger underpinnings, the changes in our sexual appetites opened new avenues of intimacy.

Life Changes,
by Choice and by Circumstance

We talked about the title of this book. If we were naming it today, would we choose the same name? Were we still on the fast track, and even if we were, was it the same fast track, or had we made changes? We agreed that the title was still appropriate, and that we would continue to live busy, fulfilling lives in which we would need to check our schedules. We also recognized that we have consciously made the decision to include in those schedules things we truly wanted to do.

We found that there were major changes in the way we live our lives now. Since we last met, two of us took leaves of absence from academic positions, providing a type of freedom we have grown to like and intend to have more of. Others of us experienced major changes in our personal relationships—a marriage entered into, relationships ended, a divorce finalized, and relationships cemented. And there were major shifts for some of us in our professional careers—a graduate degree earned, resignations rendered, retirement contemplated, professional goals reassessed, and a job change and move to another part of the country. Though some of the changes we experienced were by force of circumstance, by and large they were the results of our conscious choices.

Cathy remains on her fast-paced career path and loves it. Since turning forty, Cathy feels she has acquired a new sense of maturity, of coming into womanhood. The economic struggles of others around her have made Cathy grateful to have a stable position, and she considers it a blessing that her job has evolved along with her—that her work continues to be creatively challenging and has been a catalyst for her personal growth. As Cathy relates, "I am still active in the breast cancer movement, but I feel I am moving to another level in my cancer journey. I am still committed to 'the cause' of breast health education and advocacy, but I see my passions changing. I feel now more like an 'elder.' My life and who I am makes sense to me. I understand what events (good and bad) have molded me into who I was before, how this has contributed to who I am now—and I live with a sense of positive anticipation of the person God is still creating me to be."

Sally rushed back to work as soon as possible after her stem-cell transplant but has since realized that her values and focus have changed. The fifteen months back at work were very stressful. The increasingly unpredictable and uncontrollable pain made it difficult for her to reliably maintain a teaching schedule. Sally relates that "the ever more negative political atmosphere at work, combined with chemo treatments, led me to realize that there is much more to living the time that is left than publishing another article or grading another set of papers." Sally has taken a leave of absence from work and is enjoying special time with her partner, Jim. They have taken a three-month trip in their motor home, which allows Sally the opportunity on pain days to take her medications and sleep and to stop in clinics along the way for chemo treatment, while also enjoying the good days. Her schedule is still very important, but now it is full of time with friends, enjoying her favorite sports, experiencing nature, and growing spiritually, rather than publishing, grading, and meetings. "The people in our lives and what we have meant to them is what is most important in the end, not the success of our careers."

Now that Carol W. has completed her master's degree program in substance abuse counseling, she is contemplating her future. "Freedom from academic restraints has initiated the thinking process about retirement from the day-to-day business world. It is evolving." Carol has learned to take advantage of her newfound ability to not always feel responsible for everyone else. "In learning to 'peel off this second skin of being everyone's mother,' I had to learn to take time to do the things I wanted to do and not feel guilty about doing so. I have no qualms now about telling people *no*; it feels good saying no and meaning it." Carol is more self-focused, something that had been completely out of character for her.

For Carol H., a long-term relationship turned into marriage just before this gathering; she turned in her letter of resignation and became an instant mom when her husband's young son chose to live with them, years after her own sons had grown up and moved away. "I found I have time to spend as a volunteer with the local hospice organization and as a counselor to other people diagnosed with cancer. I now enjoy God's many wondrous gifts: my disease-free life, my loving and supportive husband, our combined children, families, and friends."

Leaving a marriage that, though not bad, was not good enough; giving up a grinding schedule in an emergency medical clinic in which she was a partner; and moving from the Midwest to the Northwest were some of the major decisions Daria made since we last met. For Daria, these were decisions made to help her embark on a more healthy way of life. "I don't know if I will die from cancer, heart disease, or something else. I'm just no longer willing to waste my time. I want off the superhighway. I want relationships that are only positive. Few people on their deathbeds wish they had spent more time at the office. That's why I chose to make changes in my life now." When Daria made the decision to leave her professional partnership, she told her colleagues, "'I don't mind working hard, but I mind dying for you. I will not give my life to the hospital. I'll work hard and do my share.' They agreed. Giving up the power and position was easy."

"I have always approached cancer like a math problem, feeling there must be an answer," Joy told us. Becoming eligible for Social Security benefits encouraged Joy to "cut back," and cutting back is not something she ever considered before. "Considering cutting back now reflects the growth I feel I have made. I no longer feel the need to be perfect. My psychiatrist even noted that I changed from saying 'my cancer' to 'when I had cancer.'" Joy is now limiting her real estate practice to only those clients she really wants to work with and spends as much time as possible with her family.

"I am still on the fast track as an attorney, but I am doing it somewhat differently than I did before my diagnosis," says Betsy. She has spent her entire adult life preparing professionally for this time, a time when she feels she has the maturity and the experience to be the kind of lawyer she always wanted to be. "My activities with the Breast Cancer Coalition have continued, although like Cathy, I find that my orientation has changed somewhat. Professionally, I have chosen to focus much of my law practice toward women's medical/legal issues. I hope that I am a role model. I take that responsibility personally. I made the decision to practice law for however long it is a workable, viable option for me." She finds business decisions are much easier to make now. As Betsy puts it, "Nothing can ever be as difficult as that time of dealing

with the diagnosis of breast cancer and the following
months of decisions and therapies."

During the time between our first meeting and this one,
Donna's focus changed dramatically. After deciding on a
stem-cell transplantation in the spring of 1994, Donna
and Mark had many other important decisions to make.
Though she planned her exit from her employment and
chose her successor, she found that these kinds of issues
were not as important as her disease progressed. Donna's
focus became getting the most out of the time she had.
Using money for a retirement that would probably never
be, Donna and Mark began their "trip of a lifetime,"
which included New Zealand, Australia, Fiji, and their
favorite place, Kauai, Hawaii. It was clear that Donna no
longer defined herself as a professional woman. In fact,
she discussed how quickly that identity left her once she
left her job. Donna wanted to be known for what was in
her heart, not for what job she'd had.

The Many Faces of Pain and Suffering

Pain and suffering are as individual as fingerprints. No
one can fully appreciate the pain and suffering another
person experiences. We talked about all the pain—physical, psychic, and emotional—and its many manifestations
that we have experienced as a part of living with cancer.

Physical and Emotional Suffering

"After I was told that the cancer had metastasized to my
brain, I made a conscious choice to have no treatment,"
Donna said. "It wasn't that hard. I think what is hard is

suffering the psychic or physical parts of advanced disease. I have had some very profound physical suffering that overpowered everything else, so the decisions we are making right now are not that difficult. We are born and have a lifetime to live to do the best we can. Life has boiled down to a real simple place right now."

Joy has also faced physical pain. "I still have pain and sometimes numbness. I am trying to eliminate pain pills, but I recently fractured my pelvis. In the past year, I have broken several bones, probably because they were the ones most weakened by the cancer."

Pain kept Sally from participating fully in our reunion, causing her to miss some sessions. Donna expressed surprise that Sally's medical team was not able to control her pain, commenting that there should be no reason we have to suffer with pain. Yet, as Sally states, "I still have intermittent pain that is resistant to effective treatment."

For others, the pain is emotional. "I feel very inadequate to deal with the depth of trauma for me personally that was associated with my diagnosis," Betsy says. "I still find it surprising even now, four years later, that I can touch those feelings and they are still so powerful and so traumatic. I consider myself as having suffered a trauma in the same way other people suffer trauma; some of that trauma still remains."

"I frequently relive the trauma, the emotional suffering, because, for me, it was documented on videotape," Cathy says. "I show portions of that video each time I make a public appearance, and it takes me right back to that time; it still makes me cry. For all of us, I think, the sense of grief is profound; the loss of our health, the loss of that innocence of not having to think about it. Because sadness and grief are so uncomfortable for most of us, I believe these feelings are often manifested as *anger*—an emotion that is more acceptable for professional women to both feel and verbalize."

Naming Our Fears

Fear is a part of living with cancer, any cancer. From the moment we noticed a lump, or saw a frown on our doctor's brow, or heard words like, "I think we should do a biopsy," we have experienced fear. Sometimes it was fear of the unknown, and sometimes the fear had a name.

For most of us, our biggest fear is of metastasis. As Betsy says, "Knowledge brings with it some ancillary baggage—ignorance is bliss. When I went for an exam to check for metastatic disease, I was only five seconds away from a well of fear and despair; I was alone."

Five years out from her diagnosis, with no signs of recurrence or metastasis, Carol W. is still filled with anxiety every time she goes for a checkup, wondering, Will this be the time that I hear bad news again? "The kernel of fear will always be tucked away in the inner recesses of my mind; it is a part of the fabric of my life, but I have not allowed it to devour me. Instead, it has empowered me in many ways."

As Carol H. says, "Fear can be immobilizing, and it can make it impossible to be peaceful or to love. One thing I try to do is to fear less. I see that in Donna. Fear is no longer a major part of my life, although, of course, I still have to deal with it. When I am frightened or angry, I walk because doing something physical always releases something in me."

"My fear is: 'How often do I have to go through this?'" Daria relates. Daria chose to take part in a clinical trial through which she received high doses of chemotherapy.

As a result, she has an increased risk of developing acute lymphocytic leukemia sometime during her life. This is one of the many issues all cancer survivors have to deal with. "Although I am fearful of my lab results at every checkup, this adds one other variable. My greatest fear, though, is that I will lose my ability to think."

"My great fear is of the future because I didn't plan to be here," Joy says, after ten years of survival. "The days when I can't do something as simple as signing a document frightens me, because I never planned for this situation."

Donna told us that strength, grace, anger, fear, and hurt will come to all of us, but that we'll get through it. Donna said, "The fears are there. When I wrote my letter telling you all of my brain metastasis, I didn't want it to elevate your fears of recurrence, but I felt like I could say it. It's hard when people look at us with fear because they're scared. I think it's the unknown, the uncertainty. It hurts to hang on to other people's fear or anxieties; I have given myself permission not to hold on to other people's fears. And fear comes and goes. I fear breaking a bone just sitting here because I have had pain that completely immobilized me. I would love to say that it doesn't, but it does. I do try not to be fearful of things that aren't important. I have realistic fears. My biggest fear was the disability and the pain with bone metastasis."

Our Health Care

A lot has happened since we met initially to talk about what it was like having breast cancer and undergoing treatment. We were then, and still are, at different points in our disease and treatment trajectories. For some of us, interactions with our health-care teams are frequent and ongoing; for others they occur only when we go in for regular checkups. Nonetheless, we all want and look for health-care providers who can meet our needs, both for quality health care and for quality of life.

Our Health Status

"Fortunately I have been problem-free postsurgery. This fifth year since diagnosis is a special marker," notes Carol W. "It signals that it is time for me to break the tamoxifen dependency cycle before possible side effects show up. I prefer depending on a healthier diet and lifestyle rather than on pills."

Carol S. relates that "I was in the midst of my therapy at our last meeting. Every couple of months since then I have told myself, and others, that my brain is returning from 'fuzz' back to normal. I have no idea how many times I've experienced these successive changes, and I still wonder if I will ever really know what 'normal' is."

Cathy is ten years out from her first diagnosis and six years out from her recurrence and mastectomy. "I still have some anxiety when it's time for my annual mammogram, but I am coping with that better than I used to," Cathy says. "I have a silicone-gel breast implant, which I want to 'update' before it gets too old. I've had no problems with it and may replace it with a similar implant— but I want *choices*, and I am keeping up with all the research and hoping that the new technology (soy-filled devices and others) will provide me with safe and effective options in another three or four years when I expect to be making that decision."

Betsy chose not to take tamoxifen and is not currently on any therapy. Cancer-free, she says, "My oncologist would have preferred that I take tamoxifen after the chemotherapy but is comfortable with my decision not to take it. Only after four years, do I not think about breast cancer every day."

Joy experienced something we all have heard about and, at some level, fear happening to us. She had begged her doctor to do a chest X ray following our reunion because she had been coughing up blood. And yet he failed to read the chest X-ray report. "He told me everything was fine on the X ray and that I should really celebrate reaching my tenth year of survival. Just months later, at another appointment, he realized that the X ray wasn't fine, that he had not even read it earlier, and that it showed an extensive tumor that encompassed almost everything in my chest, including my lungs and bronchi. . . . I had a series of radiation treatments to my chest area to reduce the size of the tumors." The radiation treatments were successful, and she has bounced back again in her inimitable way, leaving her physicians shaking their heads in amazement at her ability to continue to beat the odds.

Although she is now considered to be cancer free, Daria is particularly cautious of her health because, along with her status as a cancer survivor, she has a long-standing heart problem. This, plus her concern about the possibility that her breast cancer might recur or that she might develop a secondary cancer as a result of her therapy, makes every physical exam and every symptom especially stressful. She now concentrates on living as healthy a lifestyle as she can, eating well, and exercising. "I have opportunities to travel and teach," she says, "two of my favorite activities."

Carol H. was not able to take chemotherapy for fear it might compromise her immune system and jeopardize her state of remission from melanoma.

Our Relationships with Our Health-Care Providers

"I want my medical team to give me options, both main-stream and alternative. I want their opinions whatever they may be. I want to be able to discuss these kinds of things with professionals and I want them to take my concerns and complaints seriously. And I want them to consider my quality-of-life issues," Betsy says. "My relationship with my oncologist is very good. She is comfortable with the decisions I make about my health care."

Carol H. relied on a team of physicians when she experienced a recurrence. As she relates, "I relied on them to deal with the preexisting melanoma. I felt that I got good advice from them."

"The missing component in many health-care professionals is compassion," says Daria. "We hear in medical school that we should treat patients like we would treat our own families, but that doesn't always happen. Good care is also about communication. Technical skill is important, but a negative personality in a fellow physician can cause me not to refer a patient to that person."

"I often thought that oncology was a difficult specialty to be in. But what better group of people to deal with than breast cancer patients," Donna quipped. "They get the gift of knowing us! The oncology nurses have been quite good. They are very honest about saying this is part of life and we will help you and your family as much as we can, but you call the shots. But it has been apparent since we made the decision not to continue with therapy that most of my doctors and nurses have pulled away emotionally. So have the oncology nurses. They all missed some excellent opportunities to teach and to learn." Donna's husband, Mark, noted later, however, that her oncologist stayed close to Donna to the end and that he was one of the last visitors Donna recognized.

"My doctor gives me so much control, though sometimes it sort of feels like I've been abandoned," Sally tells us. She has essentially been told to set her own schedule. "My doctor is just wonderful at letting me have control. She has worked hard at helping me to not let cancer control my life. She's glad we are traveling, skiing, and having fun."

Death and Dying

With Donna initiating the discussion, we talked about the vernacular of cancer. Are we *survivors,* as many people with cancer like to call themselves? When do you become a survivor and when do you stop being a survivor? Though not a bad term, several of us didn't feel that the word fit our experience. Donna noted that when you are dying you are no longer seen as, nor feel like, a survivor.

We talked about the idea of fighting cancer. Donna said she didn't feel like a fighter herself and commented, "I read the obituaries and, in every case [living with cancer] is called a courageous battle. The metaphors of battle and fighting are across the board in the lay press." There are many warlike, militaristic terms—the fight against, the battle with, the war against, kill, destroy, victim—that are commonly associated with cancer. Some of us feel comfortable using these terms, though others feel strongly that they are not appropriate. Donna described herself as a conscientious objector when talking about the breast cancer that was a part of her body, and she carefully worded her own obituary to exclude any use of militaristic terms.

"I deal with a lot of death in my role as a physician, and it's still hard, even though it is a part of life," Daria explains. "People come into the emergency room near death, and I ask them what do they want to tell their loved ones and I write it down for them. I see the way different people die and I believe that we have a gift if we know that it is coming. It's a burden too."

"Someone said that we die the way we live," Sally relates. "We can look at the way we handle things in life as the way we will handle death. I try hard to listen to my inner voice. God will provide me with whatever death I need. I will accept whatever death comes. My spirituality has allowed me to feel that."

Cathy says, "I worry much more about my mother's death and how I will cope with that loss someday than I do about my own. I worry too much how my death would impact her and my brothers. But then I remember that my father died suddenly while still in his forties, and God saw us all through that crisis—and now I am even able to understand some of the reasons why he died so young. I am sure I will be capable of dealing with death meaningfully, in whatever form it comes, because I believe in the immortality of my spirit and in a loving God who has always been there for me when I needed him."

For Betsy, death is incomprehensible. "No one ever wants to really know how much time is left," she says. "I have an aunt who is ninety-nine. She believes in the afterlife. She has been praying for ten years to die. She is tired of hanging on. She wants to 'go home.' I feel like I will die of cancer because of my family history. I feel like it will be bone cancer. I will be the most surprised person if I die of a heart attack. I don't think that is fatalistic but simply what will happen."

"We have no control, for the most part, over what happens after a cancer diagnosis," Carol W. believes. "I have been concentrating on doing what is necessary every day to make my life more worthwhile. Donna's situation and the deaths of several friends from cancer since my diagnosis compel me not to waste my time on unproductive, unrewarding activities, because each day is preparatory for my eternity, which is only a breath away."

"We give each other as breast cancer survivors permission to handle our initial grief the best we can," Donna explained. "We also need to give people in death permission to deal with it the best they can. We expect a lot from people at the transition of death. People are very interested in death and dying. I have acquaintances who want to talk to me about it. But I don't think we should be waiting for the event of death to learn something."

Donna felt very strongly about her approaching death—how it was to take place, what she needed to take care of before she died, what she wanted to happen after she died, and the people and places she still needed to see. "I've written my own obituary," Donna told us. "I wrote that my death was from complications of breast cancer. I want breast cancer in the obituary because I want it to reflect that breast cancer is killing women."

Up to a point, Donna felt that the people around her were in it with her, but as the cancer spread throughout her body, and she began hospice care at home, she began to feel isolated. "I have people every day who talk to me as if I've already gone," Donna related. Mark tells us that in her journal following the reunion, Donna said of him, "It was as though he was turning one way, and I was turning another." She also said of us in her journal, "Don't they realize that they are dying, too?" She said she appreciated all the support she got on her journey but recognized that she would have to take the final steps alone. "I don't know what else to say," Donna told us, "except have a good day and make the most of it, and drink a glass for me."

Donna Cederberg died on June 4, 1995.

Our Stories Continue

How we handle what is ahead of us has been, and will continue to be, defined by who we are and what we believe. We will continue to use the skills that work, to evolve new skills, and to make the decisions we need to make.

What we give each other are inspiration, support, love, and respect, and we know that, though separated by physical distance, the special bond we share will always be there. We chose the title of this chapter because we know that, regardless of what happens to any one of us, we will never truly say good-bye, only *till we meet again.*

Afterword

It is fitting that this afterword be written by Innovative Medical Education Consortium (IMEC). The concept for this book was born of work IMEC conducted with breast cancer survivors in 1992, and IMEC proudly published the first edition of *Breast Cancer? Let Me Check My Schedule!* We have come full circle.

Breast cancer is a truly devastating disease. But the human capacity to persevere through extraordinary difficulties reaches and teaches many people beyond the family members and friends of the individual with cancer. To that, these women are a true testament.

We would like to tell you of the tremendous impact that our involvement with these women and the development of this book has had on us, as individuals and as a company.

When we first met, the women whose stories you have just read were all in a mode of self-discovery brought on by their breast cancer. Like many people, they rarely took the time for in-depth introspection until they faced their own mortality head-on upon hearing the diagnosis of breast cancer.

Whether at home in their daily lives or at the two retreats we held, these women continued to evaluate, reevaluate, and question themselves. What's important in my life? Will those things still be important to me in the long term? And what if there is no long term? Perhaps it was this self-questioning and their willingness to share their answers that drew us to them as people and why we have maintained relationships with them that go far beyond that of publishers and authors (for they truly are the authors of the book) to that of friends.

We feel fortunate to have been allowed into their circle of friendship—the bond they have with each other. This bond is very apparent in the many phone calls, visits, dinners, and letters we share. We talk of life—of living, loving, family, and friends. It was this sharing that was the catalyst for bringing them together for the second time just weeks before Donna's death on June 4, 1995.

Life goes on—

Cathy maintains her commitment to continued personal growth and awareness through her family, her work, and her relationship with God. By following her desire and leaving the hectic business world behind, Carol H. has the time to do the things that make her soul smile. Carol S. was able to bring some closure to important areas in her life with the completion of her book; she has since resumed her professorial position at UC Berkeley. Amy maintains her busy schedule of advocacy work while meeting the incredible physical challenges she faces as the result of a serious automobile accident she suffered in 1996. The changes Daria made, in her work, her personal relationships, and even where she lives have revitalized her and given her a renewed enjoyment of life. Betsy continues to live in New York City and to practice the kind of law she always dreamed of. And Carol W. has retired from her "professional" career to a new life of giving and volunteering.

Unfortunately, the disease goes on as well—

Though unable to completely control her enduring pain from metastatic, though stable, disease, Sally continues to wrestle precious, intermittent, pain-free days out of life so that she and her partner can do the two things they enjoy most: skiing and scuba diving. And Joy is, once again, fighting metastatic disease. She entered hospice care in the last half of 1996, though she was released from their care in early 1997 because, as she puts it, "I really don't know how to do this dying thing." She was able to enjoy a grand sixtieth birthday celebration in March 1997. The party, hosted by her children, was attended by more than a hundred family and friends, as well as a number of us involved with this book, including Daria and Cathy. Shortly after the party, Joy called to say that she was starting another round of chemotherapy. Since she didn't "die on schedule," she has decided to get on with living, against unbelievable odds. Behind this sheer tenacity, however, dwells a gentle and vulnerable soul. (Joy Edwards died on May 25, 1997, after this was written.)

To know each of these ten incredible women is a gift beyond measuring. We found more than we could have ever hoped for—friends to love and cherish forever, in life and in memory. We hope you, too, have found something special by reading their stories.

Innovative Medical Education Consortium

About the Book and Editors

THEY COME FROM DIFFERENT BACKGROUNDS and from professions as varied as medicine, education, and entertainment, but these ten women share one thing in common: They all have breast cancer. This book describes their experiences, exploring their initial fear, rage, and uncertainty, and reveals how each eventually coped, in her own way, with her diagnosis.

In addition to these inspiring stories, *Breast Cancer? Let Me Check My Schedule!* features step-by-step tactics to help women handle the emotional, sexual, and occupational impact of this disease and includes practical information on finding proper health care, locating support groups, and more. It is a vital resource for women who aren't ready to relinquish control of their lives to cancer.

Peggy McCarthy is the founder and executive director of Innovative Medical Education Consortium (IMEC), a nonprofit medical organization dedicated to meeting the needs of underserved populations. She also serves on the board of several cancer organizations. **Jo An Loren,** editor-in-chief of IMEC, has been a science and health administrator since the 1970s.